BARBARA CASS-BEGGS

YOUR BABY NEEDS MUSIC

WARD LOCK LIMITED · LONDON

This book is dedicated with love and thanks to Penny and Nicholas Geer of Vancouver and their three children — Samantha, Jill, and Noel — who have all contributed to my research.

Douglas & McIntyre Ltd.
1875 Welch Street
North Vancouver, British Columbia

ISBN 0-88894-213-3

Published in Great Britain in 1979 by

Ward Lock Limited
116, Baker Street
London W1M 2BB

A Pentos Company

ISBN 0-7063-5900-3

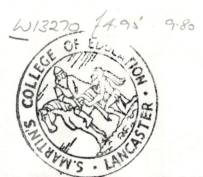

"Prayer Before Birth" on page 11 is reprinted from *Collected Poems* by Louis MacNeice, 1966, by kind permission of Faber and Faber Ltd., London, England; also from *The Collected Poems* by Louis MacNeice, edited by E. R. Dodds, copyright © The Estate of Louis MacNeice, 1966. Reprinted by permission of Oxford University Press, Inc., New York. "For a Child Expected" on page 90 is from *Nine Bright Shiners* by Anne Ridler, Faber and Faber Ltd. London, England, and from *Collected Poems of Anne Ridler*, copyright © Anne Ridler 1961, Macmillan Publishing Co., Inc., New York. The first verse of "Patapan" on page 119 from *The Oxford Book of Carols,* is reprinted with permission of Oxford University Press. London, England. An excerpt on page 134 from *The Children's Bells* by Eleanor Farjeon is used with the permission of the publisher, David Higham Associates Limited, London, England.

Jacket photograph by Christopher McFarlane
Music setting by The Empire Music Company Limited
Printed and bound in Canada by the Hunter Rose Company Ltd.

Contents

Introduction 4

    Notes on Breathing & Singing 7

    Voice Exercises 8

1 / Before Birth 11

2 / The New Born Baby 13

    Music: First Exercise; Croons; Lullabies 17

3 / At Three Months 28

4 / From Three to Six Months 31

    Music: Body Rhymes & Chants; Bath Songs;

    Leg Riding & Knee Bouncing Songs & Rhymes;

    Dandling Songs; Play Songs 33

5 / From Six Months to a Year 49

6 / From Twelve to Eighteen Months 52

    Music: Nursery Rhymes; Action Songs;

       Finger & Leg Rhymes; Chants 58

7 / From Eighteen Months to Two Years 72

    Music: Rhythms; Action Songs; Singing Games;

    Dressing Songs; Chants & Rhymes 78

8 / The Two-Year-Old 90

    Music: Outdoor Songs; Indoor Songs; Outdoor

    Play; Indoor Play (Hand & Finger Rhymes);

    Pitch & Rhythm Songs; Dressing Ryhmes 96

9 / Making Musical Instruments 119

10 / Running a Music Group 123

11 / Suggested Records for Children 128

12 / Suggested Music for Mothers 131

13 / Suggested Reading 134

Acknowledgements 137

Music Credits 137

Author's References 139

Index of Music (First Lines) 142

Introduction

A good deal of attention has been paid in the past to the musical needs of the child from two to six years of age, but little to those of the neonate (birth to one month) and the baby (one month to two years); yet, as research has proved, these are the most important learning periods in a child's life.

Until fairly recently we thought that during its first two years an infant's needs were mainly physical. We now know that infants in institutions whose physical needs alone are met do not become healthy and happy babies. Infants are not just recipients but are involved in life and need individual attention and loving care. Their environment must provide freedom and variety to stimulate their senses, for the growth of the body and the mind are dependent on each other and on such stimulation.

It may seem far-fetched, but music is almost essential in that environment if you want to help your child's body and mind to develop well. Zoltán Kodály, the famous composer who spent so much time working with children, showed clearly how music not only gives children pleasure, but also improves their ability to concentrate, which enables them to make the most of their intelligence. The ability to discriminate, so important in learning, is heightened with musical training. The spontaneous movements that strengthen the baby's body and are necessary steps to sensory control are encouraged by the rhythms of music.

Learning music which they enjoy has helped disadvantaged pre-schoolers to "catch up" with other children through feeling successful in their musical participation. Mentally disturbed children have been able to communicate better and be more at ease with others through their participation in music.

Babies absorb sound, speech, and music very early, and when they are about twenty-four days old they can discriminate quite small changes in rhythms; at one month, infants can recognize family members by their voices, and begin to imitate sounds; by six months they can discriminate sounds according to loudness, pitch, and "timbre" (tone colour or quality of sound), and a three-month-old baby can carry on a "lalling" conversation with obvious enjoyment. A

4

five-month-old baby has recognized a musical composition as soon as she heard any part of it after she had been exposed to it daily. A baby is born with a pre-programmed ability to speak, but because this ability needs to be triggered and cultivated before it can function, the baby needs sound, and especially speech, which forms a major strand in her whole learning process.

Although the centres of music and speech are located in different parts of the brain, we know that singing helps speech, and of course croonings and chantings are closer to speech than to singing. Croonings — sounds like "there, there," "bye bye," or just hummings of comfort — and lullabies — extensions of croonings and usually accompanied by rocking — are important, for they give pleasure and a sense of security to the baby. In addition, they provide the first steps on your baby's long road in learning and will help her to speak and to understand speech.

Most healthy babies develop in the same way at the same ages, so this book is divided into age groupings with appropriate music for each age. But children, like adults, do not learn at *exactly* the same rate and in exactly the same way: some learn more quickly by seeing, some by hearing, others by touching; some babies are very active from birth, whereas others are more passive. So you must adapt the organization of the book to suit your babies. Because our language provides no word to include both male and female, in this book "she" stands for both male and female.

The croonings, lullabies and other musical and spoken material have been selected wherever possible from "folk" sources — songs and verses made up by ordinary people, often mothers, about ordinary things, which have been sung or recited for hundreds of years because they are musically or rhythmically enjoyable. You will recognize many of them and they may remind you of others which you heard as a child. The songs are simple to sing and though you may not like the sound of your voice very much, the baby will. No baby needs a "professional" singer, and the more you sing, the better you will sing. Babies thrive on their father's attention, so encourage him to sing too.

Music can be as simple as rocking the baby, humming a tune, tapping a stick or shaking a rattle, switching on the radio or playing a record. Of course, if you can read music or play an instrument, you can do even more; but just as you don't need to be a mathematician to teach your children to count, you don't have to be a musician to provide music for your baby.

If you practised natural childbirth exercises during pregnancy you will have already learned the importance of breathing, which will aid you in singing. To help those who have not taken pre-natal natural or controlled childbirth classes, some simple breathing exercises have been included at the end of this introduction.

The regularity with which you provide music for your baby is as important as the quality of the sound; it is not good enough to play a record when you happen to remember, and it does not help to have a radio playing all the time. Obvious times to sing to the baby are when she is being changed, dressed, or bathed. The wake-up period after a morning or afternoon nap is another good time, and of course your baby needs a lullaby at bedtime. But do have regular times for music, times when you too can relax and share the experience with your baby.

The period of infancy and babyhood is all too short, as the opening song indicates, and some parents, particularly those who do not think they are musical, may feel that there is not enough time for them to do an adequate job. It is surprising, however, how much you can accomplish musically and how easy it is once you realize that music is a natural part of everyone in the sense that we all have a feeling for rhythm, we all enjoy melodies and shapes, and we all desire to communicate.

So enjoy these songs and rhymes with your baby. Begin now, even if your child is not yet born, and if you have any problems, your baby will be delighted to help, for having been conditioned to rhythm and sound while in the womb she will be "naturally" musical.

Although in this book I have kept the baby's parents in the forefront, I hope that those who work with infants will also find it useful. Dr. William Fowler, an authority on day care practice in Canada, stresses the importance of accompanying all care routines with games, songs, and stories, which will encourage the baby to respond, and urges the daily playing of music, for it enriches almost all free play activities in a delightful way.

Day care centres and the like have made little use of music, partly because it is only now being recognized how much music can contribute to the baby, and partly because musical material for the infant has not been readily available. The aim of this book is to provide such material, and to suggest other sources where suitable material can be found.

Notes on Breathing and Singing

Stand or sit with your back straight and take a deep breath, expanding your rib cage and diaphragm without lifting your shoulders. Breathe in slowly, counting to four, then breathe out, counting to four. As you breathe out, try to control your breath so that it does not come out in a rush. Notice that your ribs expand at the back as well as at the sides.

When you sing, open your mouth and use your tongue, lips and, when you sing an ''ee'' sound, even your teeth. When you sustain a note and almost all the air in your lungs has been expelled, there is still some air that you can use, but only if you do not let your chest sag. Your tongue will have a tendency to rise when you are singing a high sound. This blocks the air into your throat, so try to keep your tongue flat. A good technique is to imagine that your breath is an inflated pillow and that your voice is bouncing on top of it, rather than sinking into it. You should not be conscious of your throat, nor sing from your throat.

To project your voice, imagine that your voice is in your head and is being projected by your breath into and then out of your mouth. Projection has nothing to do with singing loudly; the softest sounds can be projected.

Thinking about singing in the right way is almost as good as actually singing, for it is, after all, our mind that tells our voice what to do. You can sing mentally while bathing or driving the car or taking a walk; breathing exercises, of course, can be practised any time. If you remember to pull in your abdomen each time you do breath exercises, you will also feel and look better.

Voice Exercises

Projection Exercise

Try to project the voice and produce a beautiful tone while singing quietly.

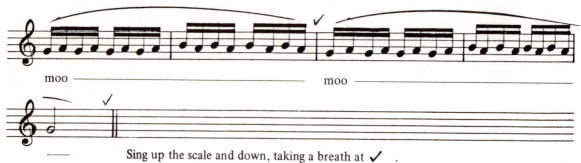

moo ———————————————————— moo ——————

Sing up the scale and down, taking a breath at ✓ .
Do not go higher than feels comfortable.

Attack Exercise

Take a breath, think the note, and sing. Try to attack the note and sing it clearly without using your throat.

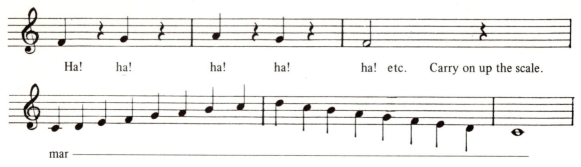

Ha!   ha!   ha!   ha!   ha! etc.   Carry on up the scale.

mar ———————————————————————————————

Continue up and down the scale.

8

Tongue Exercise   To help make your tongue free and comfortable

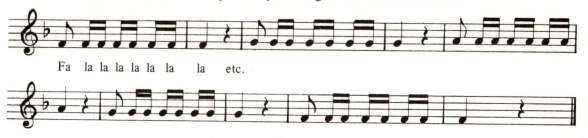

Fa la la la la la la la etc.

Jaw Exercise   To help keep your chin and bottom jaw free and comfortable

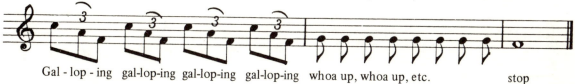

Gal - lop - ing gal-lop-ing gal-lop-ing gal-lop-ing whoa up, whoa up, etc. stop

Mouth Exercise
To help keep your mouth open, your tongue flat and your voice above your breath

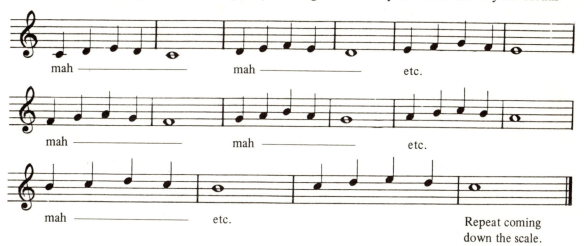

mah —————————— mah —————————— etc.

mah —————————— mah —————————— etc.

mah —————————— etc. Repeat coming down the scale.

The "m" is necessary to bring the voice forward and to make use of the lips. Try this exercise using different vowels: moo, mo, mi, mee, may, mar.

9

Turn Around

Words and music by Malvina Reynolds

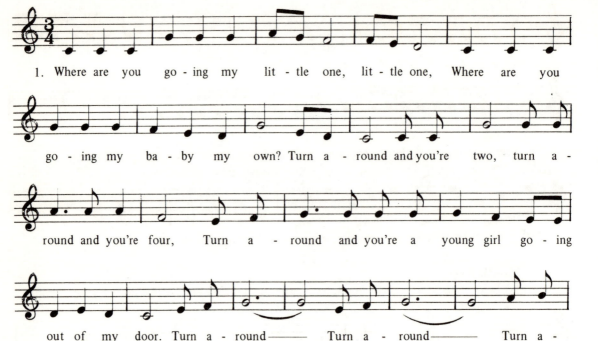

1. Where are you go - ing my lit - tle one, lit - tle one, Where are you go - ing my ba - by my own? Turn a - round and you're two, turn a - round and you're four, Turn a - round and you're a young girl go - ing out of my door. Turn a - round —— Turn a - round —— Turn a - round and you're a young girl go - ing out of my door.

2. Where are you going, my little one, little one,
   Little dirndls and petticoats, where have you gone?
   Turn around and you're tiny, turn around and you're grown,
   Turn around and you're a young wife with babes of your own.
   Turn around, turn around, turn around and you're a young wife
   with babes of your own.

10

1 / Before Birth

I am not yet born; provide me
With water to dandle me, grass to grow for me, trees to talk
  to me, sky to sing to me, birds and a white light
    in the back of my mind to guide me.

Louis MacNeice
(from ''Prayer Before Birth'')

During pregnancy, even if you suffer considerable discomfort, you will be feeling rather pleased with yourself and willing to do all the things suggested by your doctor to help you and the baby, such as keeping to a healthy diet, and getting enough rest and exercise. I have one more suggestion to make: spend some time listening to music, in the knowledge that music can increase not only your sense of well-being but also that of your baby. Music can stimulate or relax you and add greatly to the enjoyment of the periods when, hopefully, you will be taking a little extra rest, and there is good evidence to show that music can stimulate or relax the foetus also.

Although we do not know exactly how music affects the foetus before birth, we do know that from the moment of conception the foetus is conditioned to rhythm through the heartbeat of the mother. By three months, when the foetus has become almost a little human being, she evolves her own rhythmic movements and, most important from the musical point of view, she can hear. (She can also distinguish between light and dark — and although this is not important musically, it is an interesting phenomenon and perhaps explains why young babies are attracted to shiny objects, for when the pregnant mother stands in bright sunlight the developing foetus would be aware of this brightness.)

A six to twelve-week-old foetus is conscious of sound vibrations, is aware of mother's voice, of loud music, and of the sound of a heavy object being dropped. These discoveries were made by placing a loudspeaker on the mother's abdomen near the head of the foetus and a small microphone within the vagina. The sounds of the heartbeat and bodily movement of the foetus, including the movement of her eyelids, were monitored.

The rhythmic conditioning of her mother's heart from conception to birth gives her a sense of security, even of happiness, for it has been proved that babies after birth sleep better, cry less, and gain weight more quickly if they continue to hear the sound of a normal heartbeat. Similarly the ticking of a clock soothes a baby, and we find this illustrated in an old Dutch lullaby where the ''great big Tick-Tock'' helps baby tó go to sleep. Music with a strong and reassuring rhythm contributes to baby's sense of comfort and security before birth and certainly to her sense of security and growing interest in music after birth.

At the three-month stage the foetus' sense of rhythm is shown by the way she swims or floats in the fluid of the amniotic sac, swallows and cries, and even hiccups. She is aware of the way her mother moves — smoothly, jerkily, quickly, slowly — and prefers smooth, slow movements because she is then supported more comfortably. The crying periods of a new born that so often occur at supper time are possibly the direct result of her mother's hurrying to get supper during the time when she was carrying the baby. This feeling for movement, which baby acquires in the womb, explains why after she is born she can recognize people by the way they hold her before she can recognize their voices or appearance.

The foetus of an anxious mother appears to make different movements in the womb from those of a tranquil mother, and these nervous movements may persist after birth as the baby grows up. Music could help here, for if a nervous mother took time to listen to music which she enjoyed, she would find it easier to relax and in turn to relax the foetus in her womb.

The period of most rapid foetal growth occurs during the last months of pregnancy, and it is thought that profound and probably lasting environmental influences take place then. We know the damage that can be done to the foetus by malnutrition and disease and I think the time will come when we will discover that a foetus may suffer by being deprived of music. It is hoped that future researchers will tell us how music can make an even more positive contribution to both mother and baby during the pre-birth period.

12

2 / The New Born Baby

"I have no name:
"I am but two days old."
What shall I call thee?
"I happy am,
"Joy is my name."
Sweet joy befall thee!

Pretty joy!
Sweet joy, but two days old,
Sweet joy I call thee;
Thou dost smile,
I sing the while,
Sweet joy befall thee!

William Blake
("Infant Joy" from Songs of Innocence)

The new born baby spends a lot of time sleeping, feeding, and eliminating, and every now and then she cries, for this is the only way she has of telling you what she wants or does not want. She could cry before she was born, but her birth cry, which was the result of her first breath of air, was something new and might well be called a "protest" cry at the discomfort of birth. This cry changes almost at once into a "communicating" cry, and a mother very quickly learns to recognize by its tone and character what it is that her baby wants. Is she hungry, frightened, uncomfortable, hurt, or merely bored? There is a distinct difference in the sound; when she is hungry there is no mistaking what she wants, for she seems to cry with her whole body and with a terrific sense of urgency.

An important means of receiving communication at this time — again one she has learned to use before birth — is her mouth, and when she wants to find out about something new, that is where she puts it. During this beginning period, what she plays with are things that can be put into her mouth, and these are therefore her natural playthings.

Every now and then she stretches, yawns, and blinks, curls up her toes, and clenches her fists. She moves a lot, and these early reflex responses — sucking, crying, moving — soon change to voluntary movements which she knows she is making. She is quite strong and at birth can grip your finger so tightly that she can support the weight of her body. You can pull her up, then let her gently down again, which is fun and at the same time exercises her muscles. She can hear and is affected by sound when she is only a day and a half old, so you can sing as you play with her in this way (see first exercise song).

All movements, including their gradual co-ordination, are important during this first period of her life, for this is how she learns: by trying to do things and by repetition until she acquires the skill she needs — groping for the nipple with her mouth and sucking the nipple; groping for an object at random; grasping an object deliberately; sucking her thumb or finger by chance, then sucking it on purpose.

During the first month or two after birth, mothers often feel apprehensive and tense, even frightened, particularly if this is a first baby. She is so tiny; will she survive? Will I be able to do the right things for her? There is little doubt that a tense mother tends to produce a tense baby. This is the time, while attending to her needs, to talk softly to her, croon or sing a lullaby. The very act of doing these things relaxes the mother, and as she relaxes, so does the baby, so that a sense of enjoyment replaces a sense of anxiety. Fathers, too, can help by assisting with the settling down periods and the changings, and a croon or two to the baby — and to the mother — is never amiss. Actually, we need not worry, for babies are vigorous, resilient little creatures who thrive on activity.

Singing and playing music to the baby can encourage her to move, for she not only enjoys making sounds but she also enjoys listening to them and will react to what makes them. By two weeks an infant expects an object to be graspable, so a rattle that sounds and looks attractive can encourage her to move and reach for it.

When a very young baby is being looked after by someone other than the mother and is denied the close, pleasurable contact of being breast-fed, she is likely to feel less secure, even if it is not obvious to those caring for her. So it is

14

especially important that she be given extra attention, with songs and gentle talking while she is fed, changed, or held.

Because the baby can distinguish between light and dark, and can enjoy bright colours and quite complicated patterns, it is a good idea to hang balls, rings, mobiles, or different shapes over her crib. Brightly coloured posters, paintings, and interestingly patterned curtains will also fascinate her, as will a lamp that throws shadows on the walls. All these will encourage her visual perception and will help to keep her happy when she is awake. It has been suggested that when the baby cries and we pick her up and put her over our shoulder that it is not only the contact and change of position which helps to stop her crying, but the fact that she is now able to see a greater variety of interesting things. She is sensitive to bright light and will often close her eyes if the light is rather bright and open them if we dim it. If she is not asleep the sound of a bell or rattle will cause her to open her eyes and if we want to settle her down she will enjoy listening to a clock ticking, or some recorded music which is restful but has a definite rhythm.

You will have discovered how much she enjoys being held in your arms and rocked and patted, so this is a natural time to sing to her, particularly if it is close to bedtime. This is also a good time to put on a record. She will hear it, though there may be no evidence of her response at this time. Perhaps more to the point, *you* will hear it, and if you choose something you enjoy and sit down and listen to it, it may provide the necessary relaxation and sense of peace that you require before you move on to do all those things which you have not had time to do while you were attending to the baby.

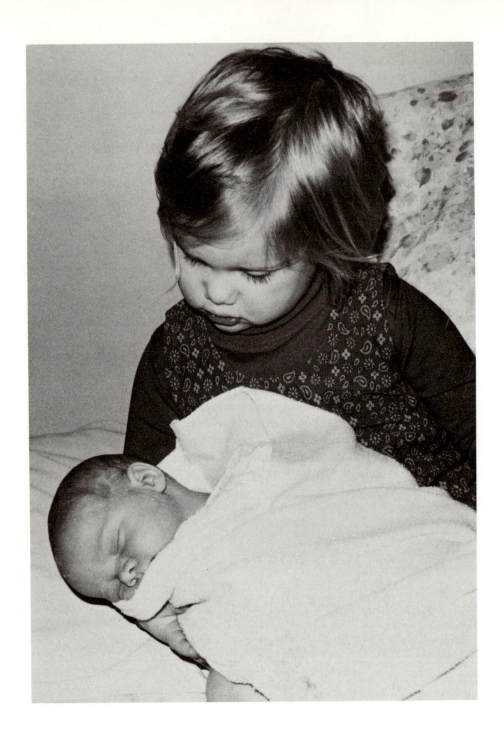

First Exercise

Now We Go Upperty Up

Words and music by Barbara Cass-Beggs

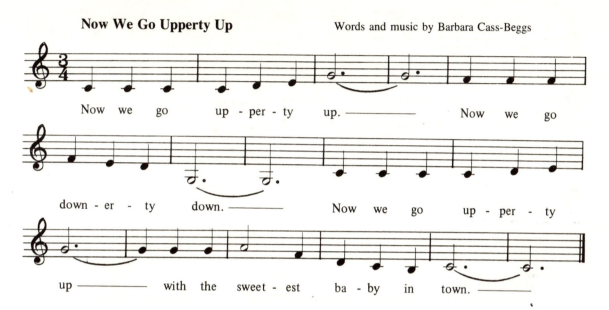

Now we go up - per - ty up. ———— Now we go down - er - ty down. ———— Now we go up - per - ty up ———— with the sweet - est ba - by in town. ————

Let baby grip a finger of each hand, then pull her up and down very gently.

Croons

Croons follow the natural rise and fall of the breath, suggesting sighing or half-speaking rather than singing. Here are examples of other people's croons. You will want to make up your own.

Bishyby

Scottish

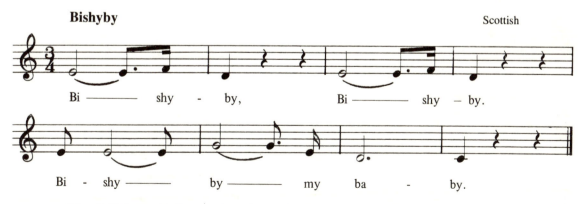

Bi ——— shy - by, Bi ——— shy - by. Bi - shy ——— by ——— my ba - by.

The "s" has a "z" sound, as in the Irish word "Husheen."

Ba Ba Baby

Micmac Indian

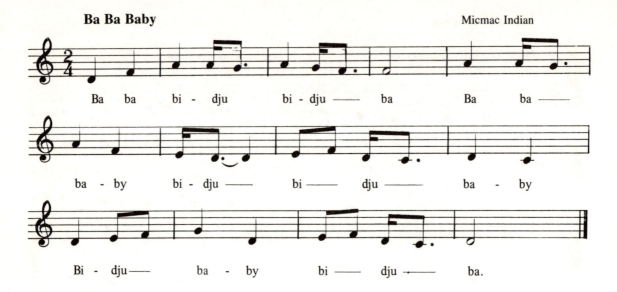

Ba ba bi - dju bi - dju — ba Ba ba —

ba - by bi - dju — bi — dju — ba - by

Bi - dju — ba - by bi — dju — ba.

Lullabies

Here are croons extended into lullabies, each one different in character, but all of which lend themselves to a rocking motion.

Hushabye Baby

English

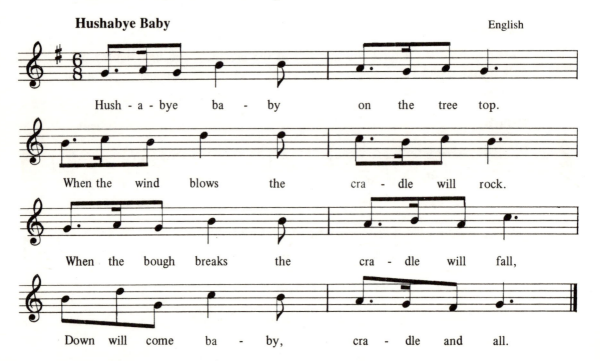

Hush - a - bye ba - by on the tree top.

When the wind blows the cra - dle will rock.

When the bough breaks the cra - dle will fall,

Down will come ba - by, cra - dle and all.

Do do

French
English words by Barbara Cass-Beggs

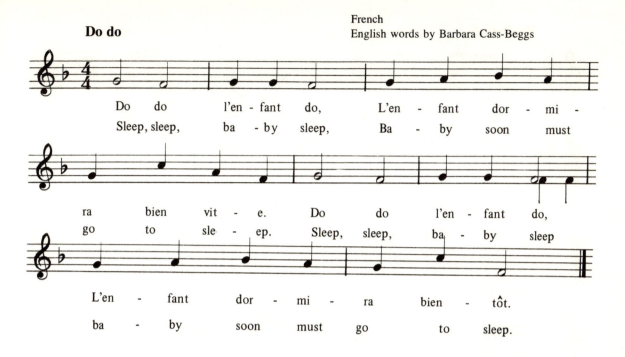

Do do l'en - fant do, L'en - fant dor - mi -
Sleep, sleep, ba - by sleep, Ba - by soon must

ra bien vit - e. Do do l'en - fant do,
go to sle - ep. Sleep, sleep, ba - by sleep

L'en - fant dor - mi - ra bien - tôt.
ba - by soon must go to sleep.

Iroquois Indian, collected by Alan Mills
English words by Alan Mills
French words by Evy Paraskevopoulos

Ho Ho Watanay

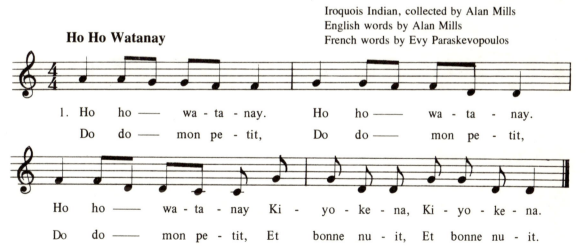

1. Ho ho —— wa - ta - nay. Ho ho —— wa - ta - nay.
Do do —— mon pe - tit, Do do —— mon pe - tit,

Ho ho —— wa - ta - nay Ki - yo - ke - na, Ki - yo - ke - na.
Do do —— mon pe - tit, Et bonne nu - it, Et bonne nu - it.

2. Sleep, sleep little one
   Sleep, sleep little one,
   Sleep, sleep little one,
   Oh go to sleep, Oh go to sleep.

3. Do do, mon petit,
   Do do, mon petit,
   Do do, mon petit,
   Et bonne nuit, et bonne nuit.

Hushabye

American

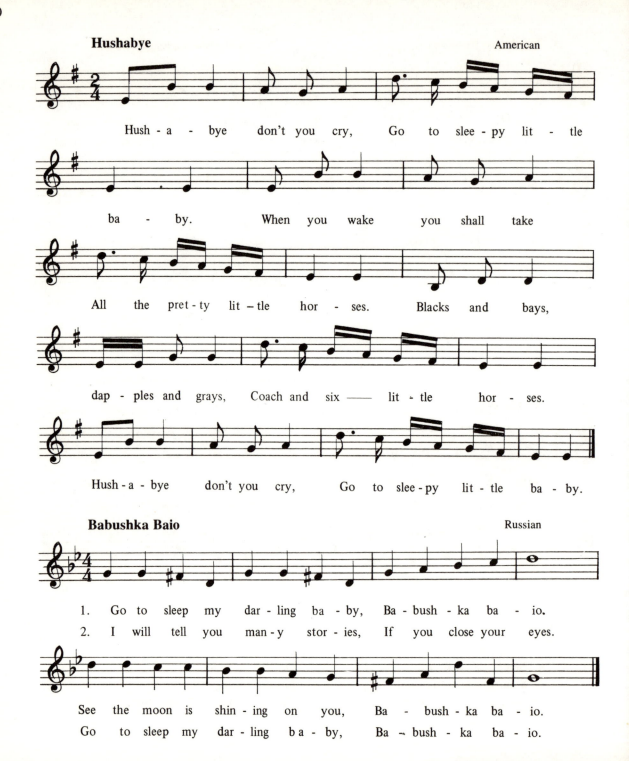

Hush - a - bye don't you cry, Go to slee - py lit – tle

ba - by. When you wake you shall take

All the pret - ty lit – tle hor - ses. Blacks and bays,

dap - ples and grays, Coach and six —— lit - tle hor - ses.

Hush - a - bye don't you cry, Go to slee - py lit - tle ba - by.

Babushka Baio

Russian

1. Go to sleep my dar - ling ba - by, Ba - bush - ka ba - io.
2. I will tell you man - y stor - ies, If you close your eyes.

See the moon is shin - ing on you, Ba - bush - ka ba - io.
Go to sleep my dar - ling ba - by, Ba - bush - ka ba - io.

Bye Baby Bunting

English

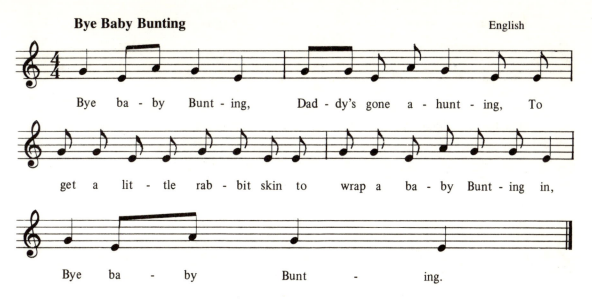

Bye ba - by Bunt - ing, Dad - dy's gone a - hunt - ing, To

get a lit - tle rab - bit skin to wrap a ba - by Bunt - ing in,

Bye ba - by Bunt - ing.

"Bunting" is a term of endearment, similar in meaning to "a plump child."

Schlaf, Kindlein, schlaf

German folk lullaby arranged by Johannes Brahms

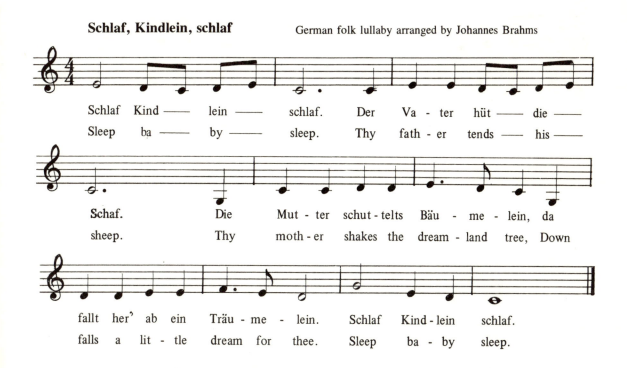

Schlaf Kind - lein schlaf. Der Va - ter hüt - die -
Sleep ba - by sleep. Thy fath - er tends - his -

Schaf. Die Mut - ter schut - telts Bäu - me - lein, da
sheep. Thy moth - er shakes the dream - land tree, Down

fallt her' ab ein Träu - me - lein. Schlaf Kind - lein schlaf.
falls a lit - tle dream for thee. Sleep ba - by sleep.

Rosiçka

Slovakian
English words by Anne Hruchair

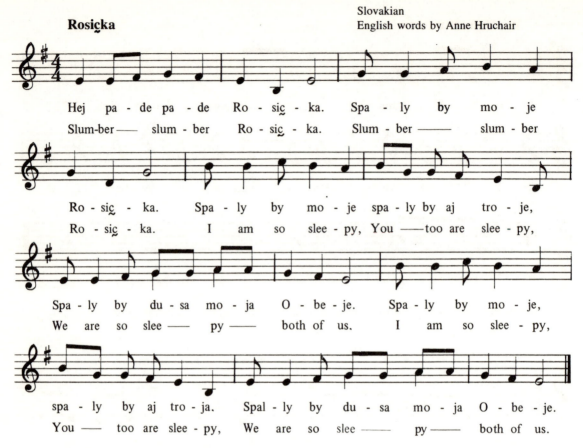

Hej pa - de pa - de Ro - siç - ka. Spa - ly by mo - je
Slum-ber —— slum - ber Ro - siç - ka. Slum - ber —— slum - ber

Ro - siç - ka. Spa - ly by mo - je spa - ly by aj tro - je,
Ro - siç - ka. I am so slee - py, You —— too are slee - py,

Spa - ly by du - sa mo - ja O - be - je. Spa - ly by mo - je,
We are so slee —— py —— both of us. I am so slee - py,

spa - ly by aj tro - ja. Spal - ly by du - sa mo - ja O - be - je.
You —— too are slee - py, We are so slee —— py —— both of us.

"Rosiçka" is a term of endearment, like "honey" or like the French term "petit chou."

Hoe laat is't?

Dutch
Words by Jaap Kumst

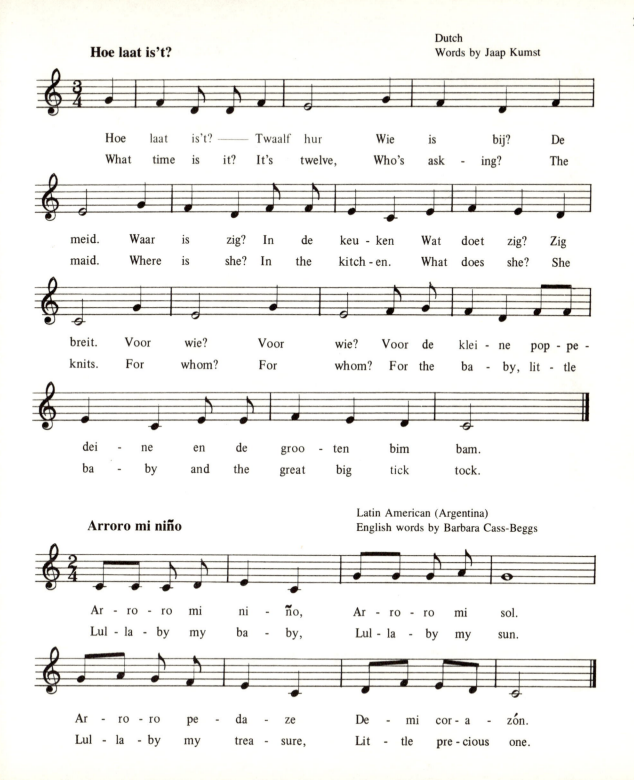

Hoe laat is't? —— Twaalf hur   Wie is bij? De
What time is it? It's twelve,   Who's ask - ing? The

meid.   Waar is zig?   In de keu - ken   Wat doet zig? Zig
maid.   Where is she?   In the kitch - en.   What does she? She

breit.   Voor wie?   Voor wie?   Voor de klei - ne pop - pe -
knits.   For whom?   For whom?   For the ba - by, lit - tle

dei - ne en de groo - ten bim bam.
ba - by and the great big tick tock.

Arroro mi niño

Latin American (Argentina)
English words by Barbara Cass-Beggs

Ar - ro - ro mi ni - ño,   Ar - ro - ro mi sol.
Lul - la - by my ba - by,   Lul - la - by my sun.

Ar - ro - ro pe - da - ze   De - mi cor - a - zón.
Lul - la - by my trea - sure,   Lit - tle pre - cious one.

Night Hymn

Melody: Eudoxia
Words by S. Baring Gould

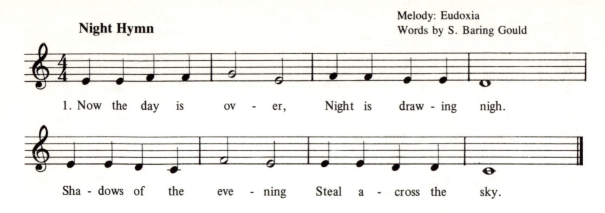

1. Now the day is ov - er, Night is draw - ing nigh.

Sha - dows of the eve - ning Steal a - cross the sky.

2. Now the darkness gathers,
   Stars begin to peep.
   Birds and beasts and flowers
   Soon will be asleep.

3. Grant to all the weary
   Calm and sweet repose
   With thy tend'rest blessing
   May our eyelids close.

Go To Sleep

Afro-American plantation song

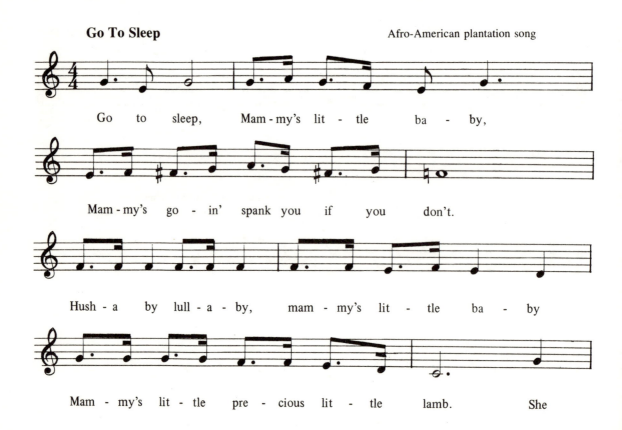

Go to sleep, Mam - my's lit - tle ba - by,

Mam - my's go - in' spank you if you don't.

Hush - a by lull - a - by, mam - my's lit - tle ba - by

Mam - my's lit - tle pre - cious lit - tle lamb. She

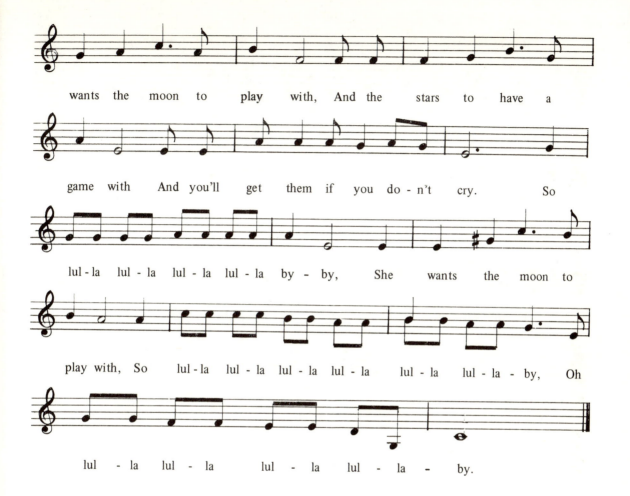

wants the moon to play with, And the stars to have a

game with And you'll get them if you do - n't cry. So

lul - la lul - la lul - la lul - la by - by, She wants the moon to

play with, So lul - la lul - la lul - la lul - la lul - la lul - la - by, Oh

lul - la lul - la lul - la lul - la - by.

Lullaby for Noel   Words and music by Penny Geer

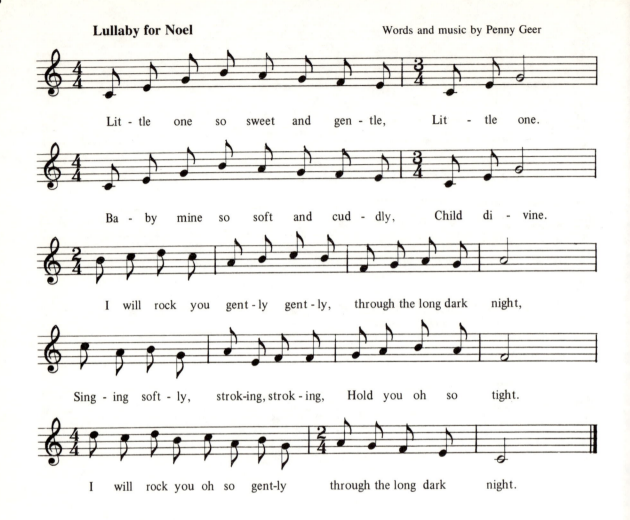

Lit - tle   one   so   sweet   and   gen - tle,   Lit - tle   one.

Ba - by   mine   so   soft   and   cud - dly,   Child   di - vine.

I   will   rock   you   gent - ly   gent - ly,   through the long dark   night,

Sing - ing   soft - ly,   strok - ing, strok - ing,   Hold   you   oh   so   tight.

I   will   rock you oh so   gent - ly   through the long dark   night.

A Blessing   English

Matthew, Mark, Luke and John
Bless the bed that I lie on.
Four angels to my bed,
Two to bottom, two to head,
Two to hear me when I pray,
Two to bear my soul away.

A Lullaby

(To be murmured until baby is asleep.)

Hush-a-ba birdie, croon, croon,
Hush-a-ba birdie, croon.
The sheep are gane to the silver wood,
And the cows are gane to the broom, broom.

And its braw milking the kye, kye,
Its braw milking the kye,
The birds are singing, the bells are ringing,
The wild deer come galloping by, by.

And hush-a-ba birdie croon, croon,
Hush-a-ba birdie croon,
The gaits are gane to the mountain hie,
And they'll no be hame till noon, noon.
And they'll no be hame till noon.

3 / At Three Months

My baby has a mottled fist,
*   My baby has a neck in creases;*
My baby kisses and is kissed,
*   For he's the very thing for kisses.*

Christina Rossetti
(from ''Sing-Song'')

By three months our baby is smiling, cooing and uttering vowel-like sounds. She listens to nonsense rhymes, recognizes the sound of her mother's voice and those of people she knows, as well as the sound of her rattle. You can help her to become increasingly aware of her hands and feet and body, and what she can do with them, by singing finger, toe, and body songs to her at changing time or bath time. When you sing or chant rhymes, be sure to enunciate the words clearly, letting her watch your mouth and lips, for your talking and singing is a valuable aid to her understanding of language.

Another way to encourage her interest in speech is to listen to the sounds she makes, then imitate them. She will love this game, and will often carry on a long ''conversation'' with you. Occasionally introduce a new sound; for example, if she babbles something like ''aa aa aa, o o o aa,'' first imitate these sounds and then say ''ba ba ba, bo bo bo ba.'' Whether she imitates you or not she will enjoy listening to you. Make your part of the game rhythmical, perhaps by clapping, and introduce new consonants such as ''ga ga ga, ba ba ba, da da da boo!'' There is really nothing new about this; people have always made noises to babies on the assumption that they like to hear them, and usually babies do. But whereas amusing or arresting sounds have their place, proper speech is equally important, even at this age; what is known as "baby talk" is unnecessary and unhelpful.

About now you could introduce a regular play time, perhaps after baby's morning or afternoon nap, when you can try all kinds of interesting experiments, such as seeing at what stage she turns her head, not because she sees you but because she hears you, or when she looks at or tries to reach for her rattle, not because she sees it but because she hears it. If you have something which makes a nice sound when it is hit or pulled (a cord that starts a music box, or a bell that jangles if it is hit or pushed), she may be persuaded to activate the sound-making object herself, and in this way she begins to discover how to influence her environment.

Around this age many infants react in fear to sudden and overly loud noises — a siren, church bells too close at hand, the sudden bang of a door. Although the unusual and sudden sound may startle her, it will not harm her hearing in any way, for sounds that can cause harm have to be continuous and louder than 85 decibels. (There is an amazing variation in the sensitivity to sound from one baby to another; some will ignore such sounds whereas others may appear positively to enjoy them.)

Baby's increasing sensitivity to sounds and her enjoyment of them can often be used to great advantage. If she is upset and screaming for no apparent physical cause, such as a stomach upset, dirty diapers, or a coming tooth, she can often be calmed by beautiful sounds, such as those made by tapping glass — especially cut glass — with a spoon, plucking the strings of a guitar, or playing a few notes on the piano. Mobiles that make attractive sounds can be set into motion. Because these are new sounds, they will attract her attention better than rocking, singing, or talking, and once she has become aware of these interesting sounds she will want to look at what makes them. By this time her crying will have died down, and life can return to normal.

Physically, the baby is now much more active. She waves her arms and legs, and kicks her feet. She is beginning to grasp with her hands, and she reaches for things that she wants to put in her mouth. Placing within her reach objects that are brightly coloured and small enough to get hold of (but large enough not to swallow) will encourage her to stretch out for them, grasp them, and manipulate them, usually by sucking or biting; if they also make a pleasant sound this is a further inducement for her to grasp them. Just as she now demonstrates more clearly what she hears and how much she can move, so we also become more aware of what she sees. She looks at a ball or a ring, glances from one object to another, and follows a moving person, particularly her mother or someone she knows, with her eyes. Place a cork board where she can see it from her cot or playpen, or from a blanket when she is on the floor, and pin pictures or bright ribbons on it. Such attractions lend themselves to the beginnings of a language program: "Look at the red ribbon . . . the pretty flower . . . the funny puppy dog," etc.

The three-month stage is a very individualistic one, and if you have twins (or if there are several infants of this age in group care), the suggestions made here, particularly those relating to language, must be carried out on a one-to-one basis. It also helps in these cases if the same person is able to carry them out, for people's voices vary and a familiar voice is easier for an infant to respond to and enjoy. Many of the songs and rhymes can accompany diaper changing and cleaning up; toys and pleasant things to look at can be available in the infants' special room. If one baby is restless, it is amazing what carrying her around will do, for she will not only enjoy the personal contact and the opportunity for an extra cuddle, but she will be able to look at many more new and exciting things. Whereas the active or demanding infant usually gets the most attention, it is actually the inactive one who needs to be picked up and played with more often. Left to themselves, inactive infants concentrate on sucking and do not reach out to explore or investigate new activities, which would not only strengthen their muscles but would also help them to become more socially responsive. Musical play can provide the necessary stimulus for these babies who without it probably will need an enrichment program by the time they are ready for nursery school.

Although recorded music — soft but rhythmic — will help to settle the infants for sleep, it can never replace a lullaby sung "live," and learning lullabies should be an important part of the training of those who plan to work with babies and young children.

In the songs and rhymes which follow, I have probably included more finger and toe and body rhymes than you are likely to use at the three-month stage; however, now is the time to learn them so that you will be ready for the next stage, which is even more time-demanding than this one.

4 / From Three to Six Months

And the babe leaps up on his mother's arm: —
  I hear, I hear, with joy I hear!

William Wordsworth
(from "Ode on Intimations of Immortality")

From three months on you will begin to feel comfortable with the baby and will want to try out a lot of new things. The baby now sits up with some support, enjoys her bath, and reaches out for those sound-making objects that you have been playing for her and letting her touch. This is the time when fragile objects are likely to get broken, and you will need sturdy, pleasant-sounding toys: a range of different-toned rattles, metal bells, wooden or metal spoons, and even small drums. The baby will want to grasp and make noises with all of these, and even though at first she finds them difficult to hold and to play with, her attempts will help to develop her co-ordination.

Because everything still finds its way to her mouth, these new toys must be safe to bite and to suck. If an object is particularly fascinating she may even try to make small creeping movements to reach it. When she is not playing with her toys she is happily discovering herself — her toes, her fingers, and her genital area.

She has become more sociable, and enjoys people and attention. She also has a growing interest in word-sounds, so that in your songs you can now ask questions such as, "Where is baby's nose? Where is mummy's nose?" This interests her because she is much more conscious of you and herself as separate persons. She turns towards you when you speak to her and may delight you by holding up her arms when she wants to be picked up; some babies make a definite "uh uh" sound when they lift their arms to be raised.

All this development means that though you will continue to sing the lullabies, and the finger, toe and body songs, you will need more activity songs because she is ready to participate in them. Play songs, like "Peek-a-Boo" and "Pat-a-Cake," can be introduced, and bath songs are sung not only to have fun in the bath, but also to help get her out of the water without too much fuss. Because all babies seem to like having the soles of their feet patted gently, putting on socks provides another good opportunity for play songs. These early foot games must always have been popular, for there are so many of them, some over a hundred years old.

It is obvious now that she listens to music and enjoys your singing. She also listens intently if you ring a bell, strike a tuning fork, or play any musical instrument. She will prefer low-pitched sounds, and high-pitched sounds of great intensity may startle her.

Dandling songs, which are songs that aim at tiring out baby before we put her to bed and sing the lullaby which she now regards as her due, come into their own at this time and "stay in" for as long as any one is prepared to go on singing them! They are rough and tumble songs which have a great appeal to fathers, for no one can tumble and throw a baby about as well as they can. "Dance to Your Daddy" is a lovely one whereas "Dance a Baby Diddy" is shorter, and less energetic, and can probably be handled by Mother. As dandling songs are very getting-out-of-breath procedures it is useful to have a number of dandling rhymes to fall back on when you are too exhausted to sing.

Because the baby is now taking an obvious interest in music, some enthusiasts feel that there must be music on the radio or on a record player all the time. The baby, however, like any adult, needs some quiet periods while she is awake, for continuous music becomes merely a background of sound to which she no longer pays attention. Our lives are based on rhythmical sequences — dark and light, sound and silence, work and play — and our baby, too, responds best to such natural rhythms.

32

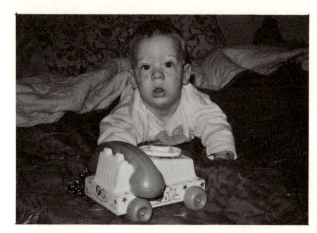

Toe Song

This Little Pig

English

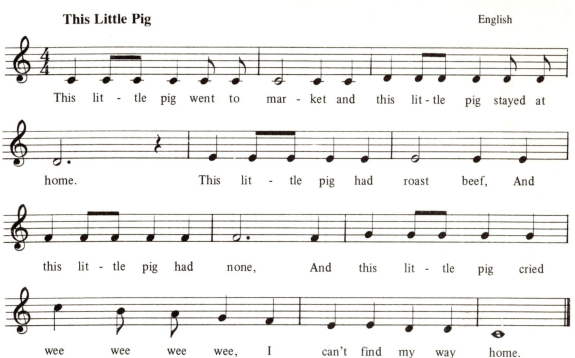

This lit - tle pig went to mar - ket and this lit - tle pig stayed at

home. This lit - tle pig had roast beef, And

this lit - tle pig had none, And this lit - tle pig cried

wee wee wee wee, I can't find my way home.

As you sing this song, touch or point to each toe, starting with baby's big one. On the last line, run your fingers up her foot and leg and body.

33

Toe Rhymes

This pig got into the barn,
This ate all the corn,
This said he wasn't well,
This said he'd go and tell,
And this said — Squeak squeak squeak,
I can't get over the barn door sill.

(As you say this rhyme, touch each toe starting with the big toe.)

See saw, Marjorie Daw,
The hen flew over the malt house.
She counted her chickens one by one,
Still she missed the little white one.
Here it is, here it is, here it is!

(At line three count each toe, pretending that you can't find the baby toe — then
 suddenly find it.)

Wee wiggie,
Poke piggie,
Tom whistle
John gristle
And old BIG GOBBLE, gobble gobble!

(Count the little toe first.)

Toe Rhymes for the Bath

This little pig had a rub-a-dub,
This little pig had a scrub-a-scrub,
This little pig-a-wig ran upstairs,
This little pig-a-wig called out Bears!
Down came the jar with a loud
Slam! Slam!
And this little pig had all the jam.

(The ''jar'' can be a sponge or your soapy hand. With each line a toe is washed.)

Let's go to the wood, says this pig,
What to do there, says that pig,
To look for my mother, says this pig,
What to do with her, says that pig,
Kiss her to death, says this pig.

(Each toe is dried as each line is said, and then there is a great hugging and kissing.)

Palm Tickling Songs

Round and Round the Garden
English

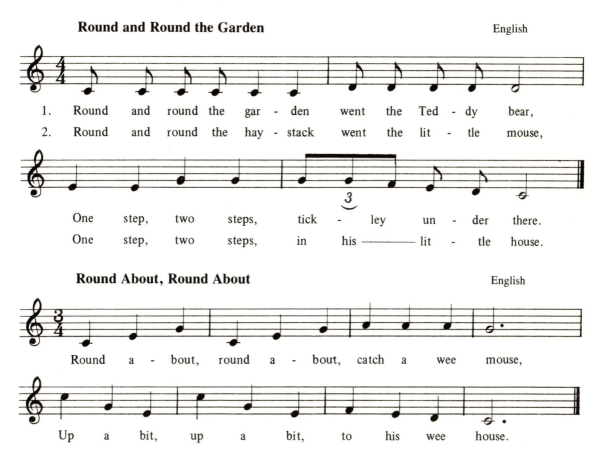

1. Round and round the gar - den went the Ted - dy bear,
2. Round and round the hay - stack went the lit - tle mouse,

One step, two steps, tick - ley un - der there.
One step, two steps, in his ——— lit - tle house.

Round About, Round About
English

Round a - bout, round a - bout, catch a wee mouse,

Up a bit, up a bit, to his wee house.

Run your finger around baby's palm, then at the last line creep up her arm and tickle her under her arm.

Finger Rhymes

This little cow eats grass,
This little cow eats hay,
This little cow looks over the hedge,
This little cow runs away,
And this BIG cow does nothing at all
But lie in the fields all day!
We'll chase her, and chase her,
And CHASE her!

(Start with the little finger.)

Round about, round about,
Here sits a hare,
In the corner of a corn field
And that's just *there*.
(close to thumb)
This little dog found her
(starting with the thumb)
This little dog ran to her
This little dog caught her
This little dog ate her
And this little dog said,
"Give me a piece please."

(Start tickling baby anywhere but reach her thumb by line 4. From then on this is a finger-touching rhyme, starting with her thumb.)

Tickling Rhymes

Adam and Eve gaed up my sleeve
To fetch me down some candy.
Adam and Eve came down my sleeve
And said there was none till Monday.

(Run your finger up and down baby's arm.)

There was a wee mouse
And he had a wee house
And he lived up there.

Then he gaed creepy-crappy,
Creepy-crappy,
And made a hole in there.

(Start tickling baby's head or nose, then finish up in her neck.)

Teeth and Tongue Rhyme

Four and twenty white kye
Standing in a stall
By came a red bull
And licked them all.

(Point to baby's teeth and tongue.)

Nose Rhyme

My mother and your mother
Went over the way,
Said your mother to my mother
It's chop-a-nose day!

(Hold baby's nose between the finger and thumb of one hand and "chop it off"
with the other.)

Foot Patting Rhymes

Pitty patty polt,
Shoe the wild colt.
Here's a nail,
There's a nail,
Pitty patty polt!

Hob, shoe, hob,
Hob, shoe, hob,
Here's a nail,
There's a nail,
And that's well shod.

Robert Barnes, fellow fine,
Can you shoe this horse of mine?
Yes, good sir, that I can,
As well as any other man.
There's a nail, and there's a prod,
And now, good sir, your horse is shod.

(Pat the soles of the baby's feet.)

Hand Songs

Tape tape   French

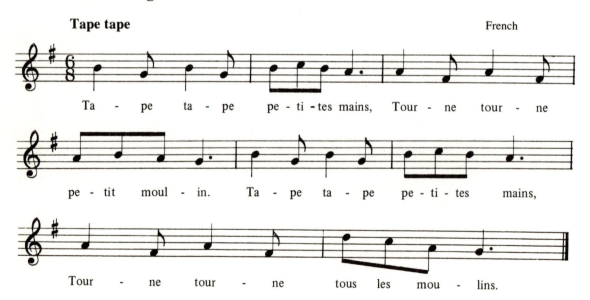

Clap baby's hands and turn them around each other like windmills.

Gai gai

French

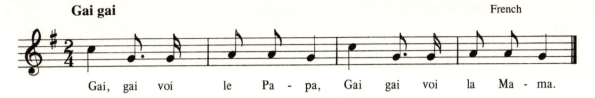

Gai, gai voi le Pa - pa, Gai gai voi la Ma - ma.

Wave baby's hands or feet to father, mother, or anyone she might wave to.

See My Fingers

English

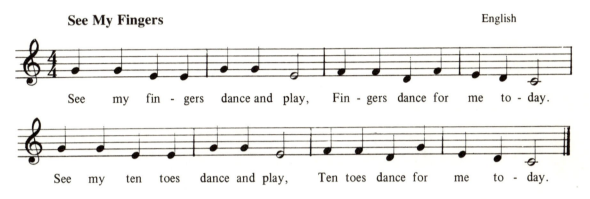

See my fin - gers dance and play, Fin - gers dance for me to - day.

See my ten toes dance and play, Ten toes dance for me to - day.

Wave baby's hands and feet to this song. Later she will be able to wiggle her own fingers and toes when you sing this song.

Bath Songs

Rub-a-dub-dub

English Nursery Rhyme

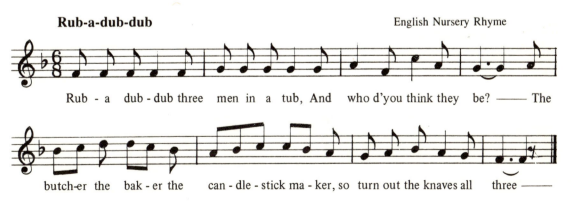

Rub - a dub - dub three men in a tub, And who d'you think they be? ——— The

butch-er the bak - er the can - dle - stick ma - ker, so turn out the knaves all three ———

To be sung when baby is in her bath. Lift her out at "so turn out the knaves all three."

Shoe the Little Horse

English

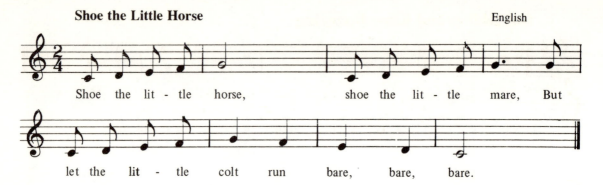

Shoe the lit - tle horse, shoe the lit - tle mare, But

let the lit - tle colt run bare, bare, bare.

As you dry the baby, pat her feet and dance them up and down. This is also a good trotting song for her when she is older.

En bâteau

French
Melody: Fais do do

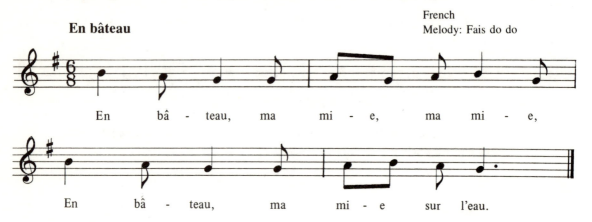

En bâ - teau, ma mi - e, ma mi - e,

En bâ - teau, ma mi - e sur l'eau.

2. Quand il fait
   de grosses vagues
   Le bâteau fait
   plout(te) dans l'eau . . .

The first verse can be sung as you dry baby after her bath. In verse 2 at "plout," open your knees and pretend to let her fall. You can also play this singing game in the bath, moving her through the water like a boat and pretending to sink her at "plout."

Leg Riding and Knee Bouncing

A Paris

French

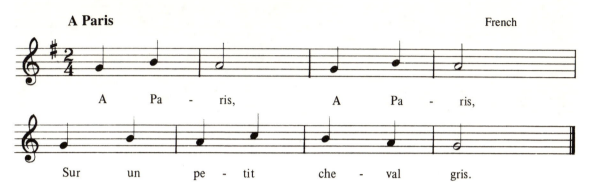

A Pa - ris, A Pa - ris,

Sur un pe - tit che - val gris.

A Rouen, A Rouen
Sur en petit cheval blanc

A Québec, A Québec
Sur la queue d'une belette

Bounce baby on your knee and add as many verses as you can find rhymes.

Au Galop

French

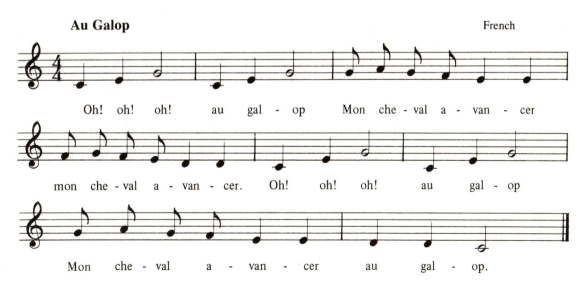

Oh! oh! oh! au gal - op Mon che - val a - van - cer

mon che - val a - van - cer. Oh! oh! oh! au gal - op

Mon che - val a - van - cer au gal - op.

Bounce baby on your knee, or make her feet gallop to the beat.

42

See-Saw-Sacradown

English Nursery Rhyme

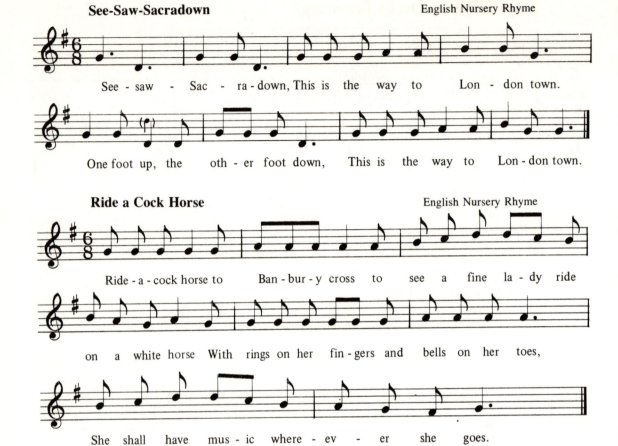

See - saw - Sac - ra - down, This is the way to Lon - don town.

One foot up, the oth - er foot down, This is the way to Lon - don town.

Ride a Cock Horse

English Nursery Rhyme

Ride - a - cock horse to Ban - bur - y cross to see a fine la - dy ride

on a white horse With rings on her fin - gers and bells on her toes,

She shall have mus - ic where - ev - er she goes.

Knee Bouncing Rhymes

To market, to market, to buy a fat pig,
Home again, home again, jiggerty jig.
To market, to market, to buy a fat hog,
Home again, home again, jiggerty job.
To market, to market, to buy a plum bun,
Home again, home again, market is done.
To market to market, to buy a pound of butter,
Home again, home again, throw it in the gutter.

~

I have a little pony, his name is Dapple Grey,
He lives down in a stable not very far away.
He goes — nimble, nimble, nimble, nimble,
Trot, trot, trot — stay behind and wait a bit
And — gallop, and gallop, and gallop away!

~

This is the way the ladies ride, nim, nim, nim;
This is the way the gentlemen ride, trim, trim, trim;
This is the way the farmers ride, trot, trot, trot, trot;
This is the way the huntsmen ride, gallop, a-gallop, a-gallop, a-gallop.

~

This is Bill Anderson,
That is Tom Sim.
Tom called Bill to fight
And fell over him.
Bill over Tom,
And Tom over Bill,
Over and over as
THEY FELL DOWN THE HILL!

(Sit baby on your lap. Take her legs by the ankles and call one Bill Anderson, the
other Tom Sim. Lift one leg over the other faster and faster until the last line,
then part your knees and allow baby to slip down between them.)

Father, Mother and Uncle John
Went to market one by one,
Father fell off!
Mother fell off!
But Uncle John went on and on . . .

(Jog baby on your knees; let her slip off to the right as Father falls off, to the left
for Mother, and trot her faster and faster for Uncle John.)

Madame de Brot

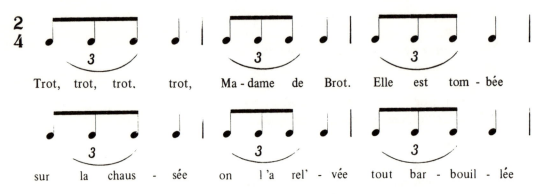

Trot the baby on your knee, then jump her up on the last line.

Chanting Rhymes

Nez cancan   French

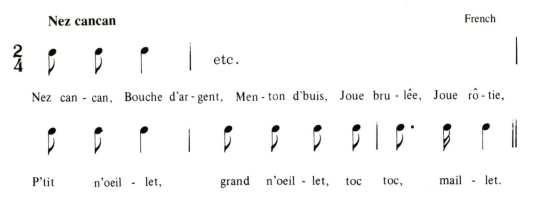

First line; touch each part of baby as you sing the word.
Second Line: touch one eye (closed), one eye (open), tap on her forehead with
    your finger.

(With the next two rhymes, touch each part of the baby as you mention it.)

Two little eyes to look around,
Two little ears to hear a sound,
One little nose to smell what's sweet,
One little mouth that likes to eat.

These are baby's fingers,
These are baby's toes,
This is baby's tummy button,
Round and round it goes.

Eye winker, Tom tinker,
Nose smeller, Mouth eater,
Chin chopper, Guzzle whopper!

(Touch each of baby's eyes, then her nose, etc. On the last line, tickle her neck.)

Knock at the door
(tap on her forehead)
Pull the bell
(pull a lock of her hair — if she has one)
Lift the latch
(lightly pinch her nose)
And walk in
(pretend to put your finger in her mouth)
Go way down the cellar and eat apples.
(tickle baby's throat)

VARIATION:

Knock at the door
(knock on her forehead)
Peep in
(raise an eyelid gently)
Lift up the latch
(touch the tip of her nose)
Walk in.
(Put your finger in her mouth)

Dandling Songs

Dance to Your Daddy

English

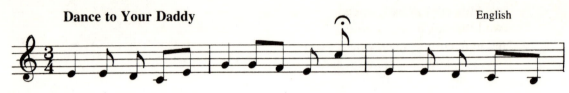

1. Dance to your dad-dy, my lit-tle lad-die, Dance to your dad-dy,
2. Dance to your dad-dy, my lit-tle lad-die, Dance to your dad-dy,

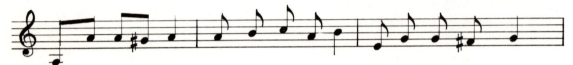

my —— lit-tle man. Thou shalt have a fish, thou shalt have a fin,
my —— lit-tle lamb. When thou art a man and fit to take a wife.

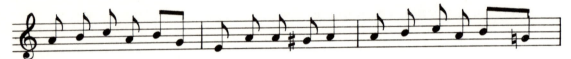

Thou shalt have a had-dock when the boats come in. Thou shalt have a cod - ling
Thou shalt choose a maid and have her all your life. She shall be your las - sie,

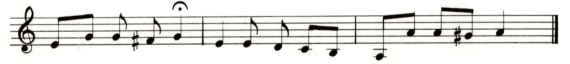

boiled —— in a pan. Dance to your dad - dy, my —— lit - tle man.
Thou shalt be her man. Dance to your dad - dy, my —— lit - tle man.

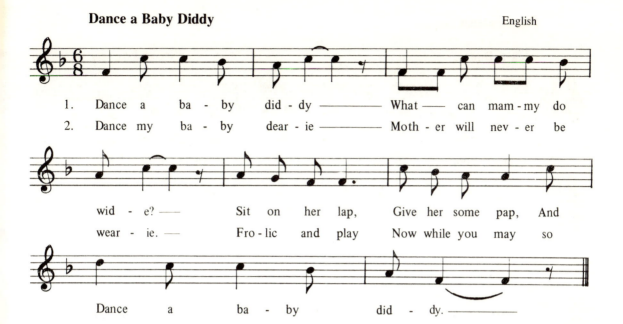

Dance a Baby Diddy

English

1. Dance a ba - by did - dy —— What — can mam - my do
2. Dance my ba - by dear - ie —— Moth - er will nev - er be

wid - e? —— Sit on her lap, Give her some pap, And
wear - ie. —— Fro - lic and play Now while you may so

Dance a ba - by did - dy. ——

Dance a ba - by did - dy. ——

Dandling Rhymes

Up and down again
On the counterpane,
High and dry and steady
Baby rides on Mammy's knee
Until her supper's ready.

Then she has her pap
On her Daddy's lap
Warm and snug and cosy.
If she's good and takes her food
She'll grow up fat and rosy.

~

Dorm dormy dormouse
Sleeps in his little house.
He won't wake up
Till supper time
And that won't be
Till half-past nine.

(This can be used if you need to wake up baby, or it can be a game to take her out
of her crib. Tickle her gently, then pick her up on the last two lines.)

Play Songs

Peek-a-Boo

English Play Song

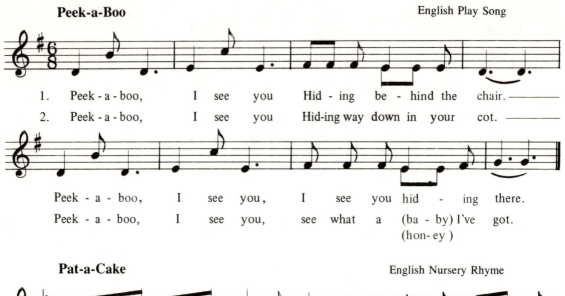

1. Peek - a - boo,   I   see   you   Hid - ing   be - hind   the   chair. —
2. Peek - a - boo,   I   see   you   Hid-ing way down   in   your   cot. —

Peek - a - boo,   I   see   you,   I   see   you hid - ing   there.
Peek - a - boo,   I   see   you,   see   what   a (ba - by) I've   got.
                                                     (hon- ey)

Pat-a-Cake

English Nursery Rhyme

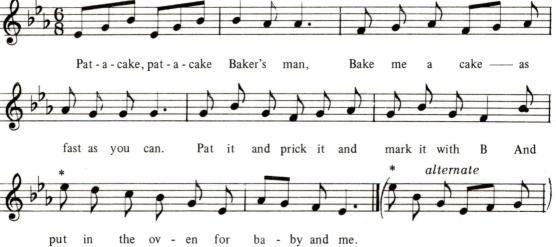

Pat - a - cake, pat - a - cake Baker's   man,   Bake   me   a   cake —— as

fast   as   you   can.   Pat   it   and   prick   it   and   mark   it   with   B   And

*

* *alternate*

put   in   the   ov - en   for   ba - by   and   me.

5 / From Six Months to a Year

Baby mine, over the land;
*   Baby mine, over the water.*
Oh, when had a mother before
*   Such a sweet – such a sweet, little daughter!*

Kate Greenaway
(from ''Baby Mine'')

At six months to a year our infant is about to become a toddler, and is probably already crawling or hitching herself around everywhere. She now responds to her name, listens to our conversations, shouts when she wants attention, and can say a few words.

She will also be pulling herself upright by holding on to anything that is handy. Not only is she sitting upright, but she is also able to roll over from her back to her stomach, so if you leave her alone, be sure she is on the floor and not on a couch or bed where she can roll off. If she is a very heavy baby she may be far less active and may not seem interested in crawling, but as long as she is kicking her legs and taking in all that goes on around her, there is nothing to worry about.

Meal times should be easier to cope with, as she can now drink from a cup and eat from a spoon, and she likes to help you hold them. Because her forefinger and thumb are partly specialized, you can add a variety of small objects to her playthings; she loves putting small objects into tins and boxes and taking them out again.

She is full of affection, loves to be hugged and kissed, knows strangers from friends, and tries to help when you dress her. She can bang two blocks together, shout and throw things, and experiences a great sense of power. We experience a great sense of her nuisance value when she throws everything out of her crib and yells for you to retrieve them, only to throw them out again.

When you sing *her* songs she likes to sing along with you, and sometimes sings by herself, especially when she is playing alone. She babbles short sentences, which sound meaningful even if they are not, and she tries to say a few words, which probably include "dada," "bye bye," "gone" or "all gone," and "there." The words "more," "no," and "ma ma" are attempted but do not always sound right, for the "n" and "m" sounds are difficult for her to manage.

She may just shake her head for "no," and is quite capable of letting you know what she wants either by her actions or by her own way of naming objects and persons. Because we usually know what she means, and because she always does, communication is managed quite well. She certainly understands our "no, no," and in fact understands far more of our speech than we may realize. For example, you might say, "I wonder where her bottle is?" and the next moment she has vanished, to return with the missing bottle.

Just as she has learned from birth about her environment through her sense of touch (her mouth, her hands and feet, and finally her whole body), so she learns sounds by hearing and then imitating them, soaking them up without needing to know what they mean. This is why it is easy for a very young child to learn a second language, for she imitates or "absorbs" and, every sound being a new experience, remembers.

When the infant babbles, she is using and practising all the basic sounds that she will use when she speaks, so her babbling is an important part of her speech development. If by six or nine months her babbling tapers off and she makes no attempt to speak, this might mean that she is not hearing properly, and you should have an ear doctor check her hearing.

The songs and rhymes that you have been singing to her are now familiar, and she is able to participate in them. They should not be dropped, for familiar things are important, but you can now add more nursery rhymes and some "pitch" games. You can sing her name with the sol-fa sounds soh and me, and she may try to imitate you. Or sing up an octave to doh', waving your arms in the air, then sing down an octave to doh,, waving your arms downwards. She will be amused and may try to sing these sounds, too. This game helps her to become aware of pitch, especially if you ask her quesions while using the sol-fa sounds.

50

		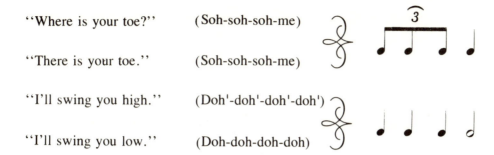
"Where is your toe?"	(Soh-soh-soh-me)	
"There is your toe."	(Soh-soh-soh-me)	
"I'll swing you high."	(Doh'-doh'-doh'-doh')	
"I'll swing you low."	(Doh-doh-doh-doh)	

If you are not familiar with tonic sol-fa, it is a method of naming the eight notes of the musical scale: doh ray me fah soh lah te doh. In this useful system the sounds are easy to sing and transposition is simple: a line placed above or below a note indicates that it should be sung an octave higher (doh') or lower (doh,). Music notation uses a single letter to represent the sol-fa notes (d = doh; r = ray, etc.).

A nursery rhyme book with music and good illustrations is a great help by the time the baby is a year old, and there are also two other books that you will find useful up to the two-and-a-half-year-old stage: *I Hear Sounds in a Children's World* by Lucille Ogle and Tina Thorburn (Collins, 1972), a book for helping your children to listen to and recognize sounds; and *The Little Singing Time* by Satis N. Coleman and Alice G. Thorne (John Day, 1940), which shows how to use simple songs to accompany all the things you do with baby and how easy it is to make up your own songs to fit different occasions.

Remember that children develop at different rates, so if you have twins or are responsible for looking after several toddlers you must not expect them to be making the same progress. One child will learn best through touching and may be slow to speak; another will listen intently and take a special delight in sounds, so often speaks early; yet another will be absorbed in exercising her body and muscles, and concentrates on movement. It is not too fanciful to suggest that the "touching" child may come to play an instrument rather well, the "listening" child may enjoy singing songs, and the "moving" child may find expression in dancing.

6 / From Twelve to Eighteen Months

A little way, more soft and sweet
*   Than fields aflower with May,*
A babe's feet, venturing, scarce complete
*   A little way.*

*   Eyes full of dawning day*
Look up for mother's eyes to meet,
*   Too blithe for song to say.*

Glad as the golden spring to greet
*   Its first live leaflet's play,*
Love, laughing, leads the little feet
*   A little way.*

A. C. Swinburne
(from "First Footsteps")

The age from twelve to eighteen months may be a rather trying one, for your toddler wants to do so much that is beyond her, and when she becomes frustrated she has no hesitation in letting you know. She wants to feed herself but is slow and messy. She helps with dressing and can take off her shoes and socks, particularly when you have just succeeded in putting them on. She is able to pull at a paper or a tablecloth with the idea of reaching something, often with disastrous results. She loves to scribble, so give her large sheets of paper and (non-poisonous) crayons and save your walls.

She is walking everywhere, and climbing upstairs but not always downstairs; she can also climb on ledges and unsafe places, so needs to be watched constantly. She is beginning to build with blocks, and likes constructive play with boxes, lids, and cubes, but does not like to play alone for more than a few minutes.

She can probably say four or five words clearly, and some toddlers have an even larger vocabulary. There is no need to worry if your toddler's speech does not fit patterns suggested for various age groupings; the important thing is her ability to communicate, not her actual articulation.

If she can walk, then a variety of musical games can be played, and if her frustrations lead to temper tantrums, you can often help her to let off steam by encouraging her to bash on a drum or stamp her feet to a drum accompaniment or a march. Naturally it is more fun if you can accompany her, and the two of you can make fascinating sounds with tone blocks, drums, a sturdy tambourine, and rhythm band bells, but none of these is as satisfying as kitchen utensils — pan lids, saucepans, spoons, or anything that she can get hold of. Because she can open drawers, nothing is safe, and she much prefers anything that is yours to anything that is hers. A wide selection of saucepan lids and other ''instruments'' strung on a clothes line low enough so that the toddler can hit them with a wooden spoon is fun in the home or day care centre.

Toddlers will enjoy ''Here We Go Round the Mulberry Bush'' with actions made to suit their latest interest — dressing, gardening, washing, etc. ''Kicking'' songs can be changed to walking or marching songs. Car and boat songs can be added because she now likes to push things around, and ''Ring-a-Round-a-Rosy'' becomes popular with its ''all fall down'' ending. Much depends on the child, but actually there is very little limitation to what is possible, so try some of the songs included in the next two sections. You will certainly want to continue with the earlier songs, but try to use them differently, for the older baby prefers action to just singing.

Because of the emphasis on activity, your toddler gets tired, often very suddenly, and just wants to be a baby again. When this happens there is nothing like a cuddle and a lullaby, which may result in sleep for her and a sudden respite for you.

If walking is still difficult — a heavy child may not get around on her feet until after eighteen months — songs like ''The Band,'' ''Clap Hands,'' ''This Is the Way,'' and the three French songs in this section can be played while she sits, and actions suggested by the songs may encourage her to be more mobile.

Two more books about music can be added at this time, both of which are also useful for two- or three-year-olds: *Making Sounds* by Gwen Clemens (Longmans Green Co., 1968) is a somewhat more sophisticated version of *I Hear;* and *Stories That Sing* by Ethel Crowinshield (Boston Music Co., 1945) contains delightful pictures painted by children with simple stories accompanying the music. You will still have to provide the singing, but the important aspect of this book is that the toddler can see the music as it is sung. Later, with your help, she can play some of these tunes on a xylophone or chime bars or even on the piano.

When you read to the toddler from a picture book, and eighteen months is not too early to start, she will see the words, just as she is seeing words everywhere — on the newspaper you read, on the tins and packages containing her food — but she will rarely see music, and unless it is drawn to her attention, she will not learn to think or read music. She should grow up realizing that music is a written as well as a "listened to" language, and that it is as easy to understand as words.

So put some simple melodies on the wall in your toddler's room. Use sol-fa as well as lines and spaces, and hang these melodies low enough so that she can touch them. You can sing or chant them while you point out the pattern and melody. You could even make a musical frieze around the room, as shown here, and all this will help her in making up her own songs when she is on her own.

Suggested Musical Frieze

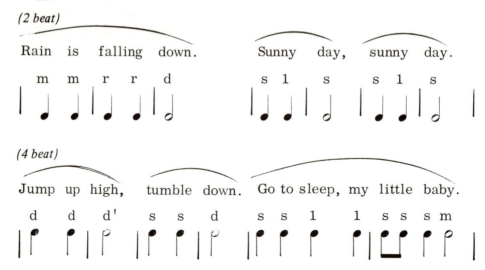

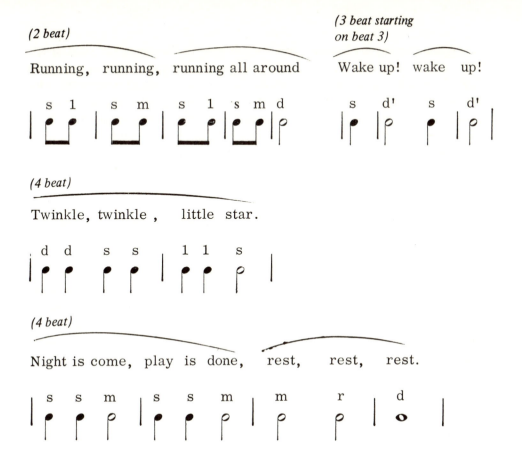

(2 beat)

Running, running, running all around

s l   s m   s l   s m d

(3 beat starting on beat 3)

Wake up! wake up!

s d'   s d'

(4 beat)

Twinkle, twinkle ,   little star.

d d   s s   l l   s

(4 beat)

Night is come, play is done, rest, rest, rest.

s s m   s s m   m   r   d

LINES AND SPACES

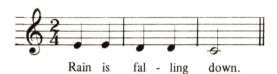

Rain is fal - ling down.

When playing rhythmical games which involve the use of the right or left hand or leg, remember that she is too young to be able to distinguish right from left: she may be about four before she has a definite preference for one hand, with the majority showing a right-hand preference. Thus in games such as "Looby Loo," it is better to say "put your foot in," not "put your *right* foot in." Right and left discrimination constitutes a subject in itself, as does motor development and its relationship to intellect, but there is no point in worrying about them during this early stage of development. What you can do is see that baby is encouraged to become aware of her body through lots of big, free, pleasurable, movements, and to explore and enjoy a variety of speech patterns and language. It is true that if we offer the baby an instrument to hold, such as a spoon, and always put it in her right hand we are unconsciously encouraging her righthand-ness. There should be no insistence, and baby must be free to change hands if she wishes.

It is through speech that baby enters the world of concepts (organized ideas) and speech appears to play an important part in identifying parts of the body, discriminating between right and left and becoming aware of dimensions of external space. This reemphasizes the importance of music, for just as music encourages free and enjoyable movement, songs encourage the enjoyment of sound, which leads to the understanding and enjoyment of speech.

When the toddler is moving to music, walking is easiest and comes first; this is followed by trotting, running, jumping and then galloping, which is a combination of walking and leaping. Skipping and hopping require considerably more co-ordination, and though some children, usually girls, can skip by four years of age, other children take longer, perhaps until they are five or even six. A two-year-old may love a skipping melody, but she will gallop, not skip to it.

Technically, a skipping melody is in compound time and usually in six/eight (in compound time each beat can be divided into three) so the notes are dotted (♩♫ or ♩♩♩). "Girls and Boys Come Out to Play" is a skipping melody. A galloping melody is usually in simple time where each beat can be divided into two, i.e. ♩♫ or ♩♩♩, but the notes can be made "jumpy" by dotting them. An example is "Charlie Is My Darling." It is possible to gallop to a six/eight beat if it is played slowly. A good way to accompany a toddler is to play on a drum, watch how she moves, and adjust the beat accordingly.

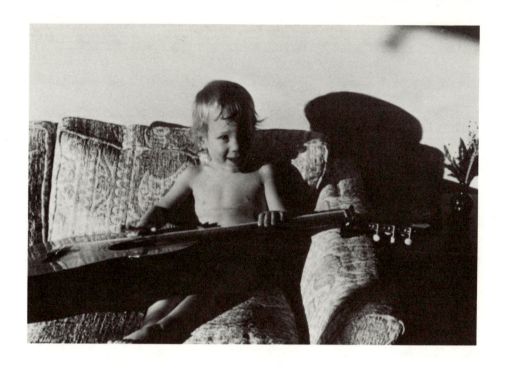

Nursery Rhymes

You will certainly not expect your baby to sing these rhymes, nor will she understand many of the words, but she will enjoy listening to these appealing folk tunes and will begin to absorb many of their details. Nursery rhymes are important at this age because they are action songs, and baby can participate in the actions with you. For example, in ''Hickory Dickory Dock'' she is the clock and your fingers are the mouse; in ''Little Miss Muffett,'' when you pretend to eat, baby will imitate you. The French rhymes are equally easy to dramatize. Whenever I sang ''There was a Lady Loved a Swine'' to my daughter at this age she would go into fits of laughter when I reached ''Hunc.'' You baby, too, will have favourites, which she will respond to and eventually choose—by finding the picture in her nursery rhyme book, singing part of the tune, or asking for a song by name.

58

Hickory Dickory Dock

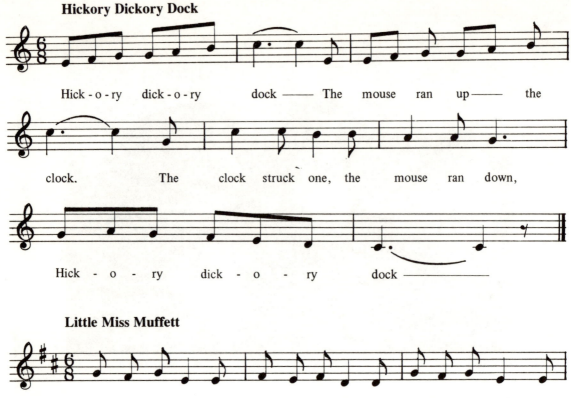

Hick - o - ry dick - o - ry dock —— The mouse ran up —— the

clock. The clock struck one, the mouse ran down,

Hick - o - ry dick - o - ry dock ——————

Little Miss Muffett

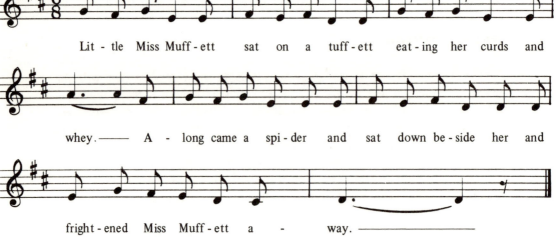

Lit - tle Miss Muff - ett sat on a tuff - ett eat - ing her curds and

whey. —— A - long came a spi - der and sat down be - side her and

fright - ened Miss Muff - ett a - way. ——————

The same melody can be used for "Little Jack Horner."

Pussycat at Court

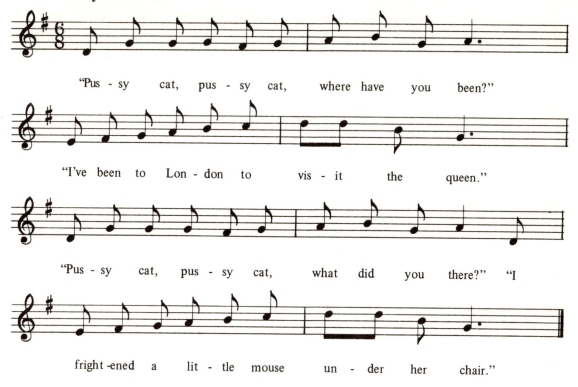

"Pus - sy cat, pus - sy cat, where have you been?"

"I've been to Lon - don to vis - it the queen."

"Pus - sy cat, pus - sy cat, what did you there?" "I

fright -ened a lit - tle mouse un - der her chair."

There Was a Lady Loved a Swine

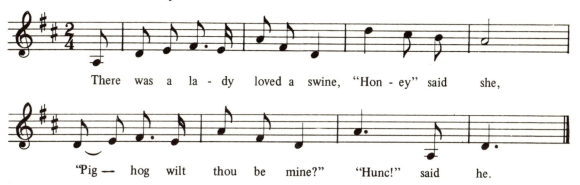

There was a la - dy loved a swine, "Hon - ey" said she,

"Pig — hog wilt thou be mine?" "Hunc!" said he.

Polly, Put the Kettle On

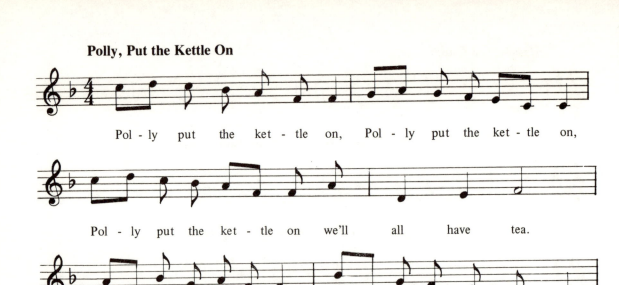

Pol - ly put the ket - tle on, Pol - ly put the ket - tle on,

Pol - ly put the ket - tle on we'll all have tea.

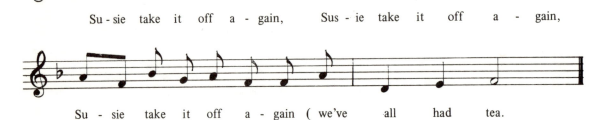

Su - sie take it off a - gain, Sus - ie take it off a - gain,

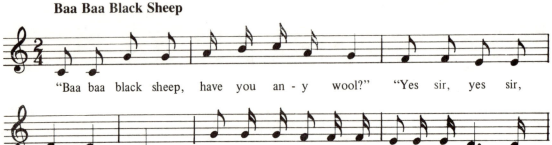

Su - sie take it off a - gain (we've all had tea.
(they've all gone home.

Baa Baa Black Sheep

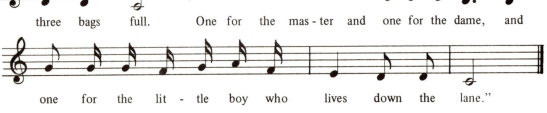

"Baa baa black sheep, have you an - y wool?" "Yes sir, yes sir,

three bags full. One for the mas - ter and one for the dame, and

one for the lit - tle boy who lives down the lane."

Jack and Jill

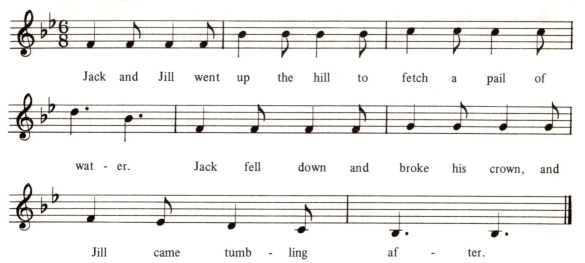

Jack and Jill went up the hill to fetch a pail of

wat - er. Jack fell down and broke his crown, and

Jill came tumb - ling af - ter.

J'aime papa

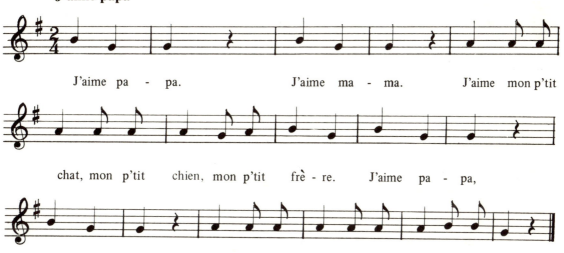

J'aime pa - pa. J'aime ma - ma. J'aime mon p'tit

chat, mon p'tit chien, mon p'tit frè - re. J'aime pa - pa,

J'aime ma - ma, J'aime grand' ma - ma et mon gros é - lé - phant.

A song for hugging.

62

Sur le pont d'Avignon

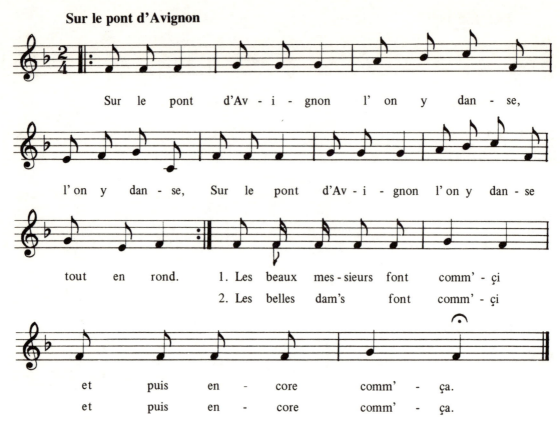

Sur le pont d'Av - i - gnon l' on y dan - se,

l' on y dan - se, Sur le pont d'Av - i - gnon l' on y dan - se

tout en rond.
1. Les beaux mes - sieurs font comm' - çi
2. Les belles dam's font comm' - çi

et puis en - core comm' - ça.
et puis en - core comm' - ça.

Move baby's arms in a dancing motion during the first part of the song. At comm'-çi and comm'-ça, nod your head to the left and to the right.

Mon papa

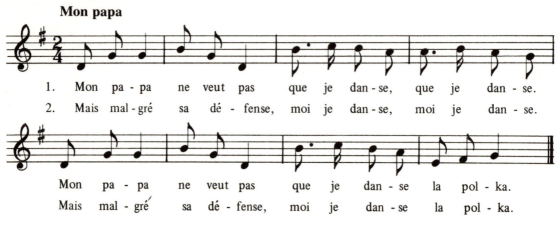

1. Mon pa - pa ne veut pas que je dan - se, que je dan - se.
2. Mais mal - gré sa dé - fense, moi je dan - se, moi je dan - se.

Mon pa - pa ne veut pas que je dan - se la pol - ka.
Mais mal - gré sa dé - fense, moi je dan - se la pol - ka.

Dance baby up and down.

Les marionettes

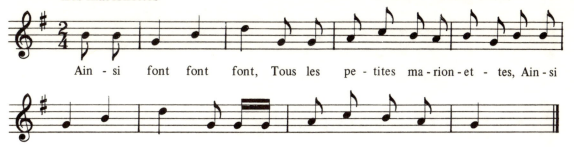

Ain - si font font font, Tous les pe - tites ma - rion - et - tes, Ain - si

font font font, trois pe - tits tours, et puis s'en vont.

Dance the baby, or dance her fingers.

Michaud

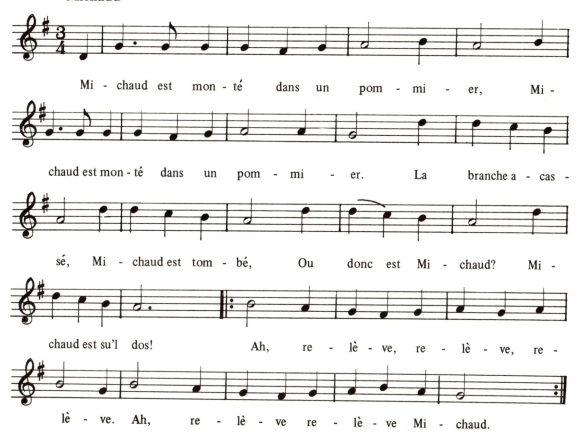

Mi - chaud est mon - té dans un pom - mi - er, Mi -

chaud est mon - té dans un pom - mi - er. La branche a - cas -

sé, Mi - chaud est tom - bé, Ou donc est Mi - chaud? Mi -

chaud est su'l dos! Ah, re - lè - ve, re - lè - ve, re -

lè - ve. Ah, re - lè - ve re - lè - ve Mi - chaud.

Monté sur un éléphant

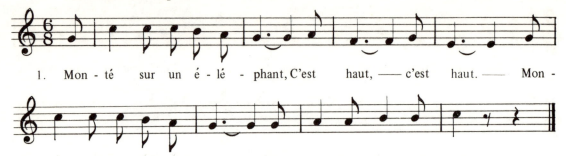

1. Mon - té   sur un é - lé - phant, C'est   haut, —— c'est   haut. —— Mon -

té   sur   un é - lé - phant, —— C'est   haut, c'est ef - fray - ant.

2. Monté sur deux éléphants, etc.

A song for lifting the baby.

Action Songs

Music: traditional

Clap Hands

Words by Barbara Cass-Beggs

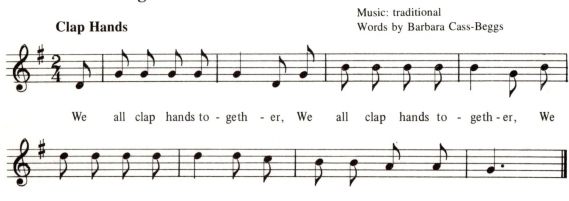

We   all clap hands to - geth - er, We   all   clap hands to - geth - er,   We

all   clap hands to - geth - er, be - cause it's fun   to   do.

(Stand up; sit down; stretch up; fall down, etc.)

Can You Kick?

Words and music by Barbara Cass-Beggs

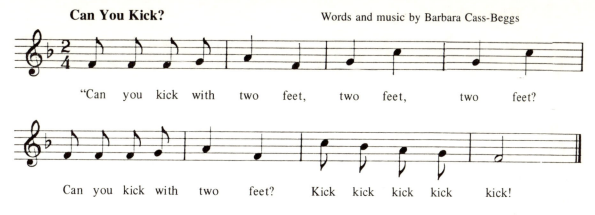

"Can you kick with two feet, two feet, two feet?

Can you kick with two feet? Kick kick kick kick kick!

Can you clap with two hands?
Can you nod with one head?
etc.

Toi toi toi

French Nursery Rhyme
Words by Evy Paraskevopoulos

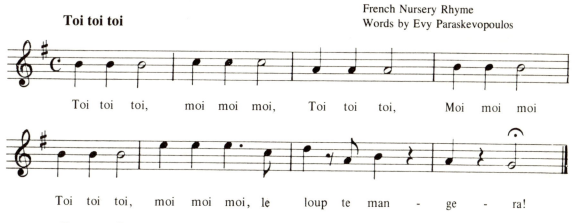

Toi toi toi, moi moi moi, Toi toi toi, Moi moi moi

Toi toi toi, moi moi moi, le loup te man - ge - ra!

Put your fingers on baby for "toi"; put baby's fingers on you for "moi"; put baby's fingers in your mouth for "le loup."

Tête épaules

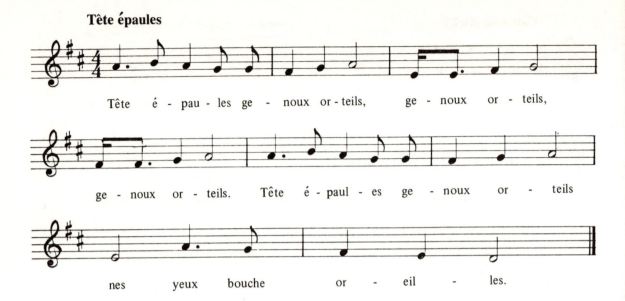

Tête é - pau - les ge - noux or - teils, ge - noux or - teils,

ge - noux or - teils. Tête é - paul - es ge - noux or - teils

nes yeux bouche or - eil - les.

An exercise song which helps baby to recognize parts of her body.

Finger Songs

Tommy Thumb

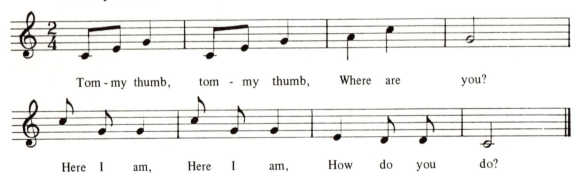

Tom - my thumb, tom - my thumb, Where are you?

Here I am, Here I am, How do you do?

Pick up baby's fingers one by one and sing a verse for each: Tommy thumb, Peter pointer, Toby tall, Ruby ring, Baby small. Then sing the song for "Fingers all" and wave the baby's hands.

Where Is Thumbkin?

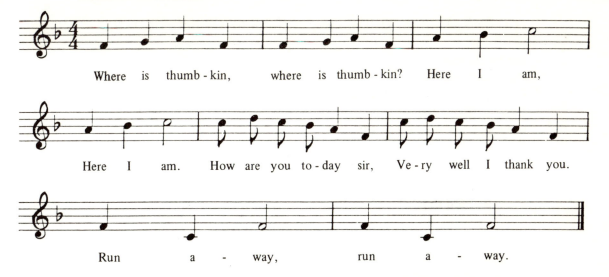

Where is thumb-kin, where is thumb-kin? Here I am,

Here I am. How are you to-day sir, Ve-ry well I thank you.

Run a - way, run a - way.

Hide your hands behind your back or under a towel, then bring them out, holding up both thumbs. At "run away," hide them again. You can sing this song using the finger names from "Tommy Thumb."

Finger Rhymes

Dance, thumbkin, dance; Dance, thumbkin, dance.
Dance you merry men every one (use all fingers)
But thumbkin he can dance alone,
Thumbkin he can dance alone.

Master Thumb is first to come,
Then Pointer steady and strong,
Then tall Man high
And just near by
The Feeble Man doth linger.
And last of all,
So neat and small,
Comes little Pinky finger.
(Touch or pick up each of baby's fingers as you say this rhyme.)

Les doigts

(To be chanted while lightly pinching each of baby's fingertips in succession.)

Sur un chemin
Passe un lapin
Celui-çi (the thumb) le decouvrit,
Celui-çi (index finger) le poursuivit,
Celui-çi (middle finger) l'attrapa,
Celui-çi (ring finger) le croqua,
Cui-cui (little finger) j'en veux un petit morceau!

Pour les cinq doigts

Par ici passa le rat,
   (glide your fingers along baby's arm)
Par ici passa la queue,
   (tickle her palm)
Celui-çi l'a vu,
   (take her thumb)
Celui-çi l'a pris,
   (take her index finger)
Celui-çi l'a roti,
   (take her middle finger)
Celui-çi l'a mange
   (take her ring finger)
Et le petit minon (take her little finger) qui n'a rien eu, dit:
   Miaou, miaou!

Amusette pour les doigts

C'est lui (the thumb) qui est alle à la chasse,
C'est lui (index finger) qui a tue le lièvre,
C'est lui (the middle finger) qui l'a fait cuire,
C'est lui (the ring finger) qui l'a mange;
   Et le petit glinglin
     (the little finger)
   Qui était au moulin,
   Disait: "Moi, j'en veux,
   J'en veux, j'en veux, j'en veux, j'en veux!"

Chants

(Touch each part of baby as you chant.)

I'll touch my chin,
　　my cheek, my chair.
I'll touch my head,
　　my heels, my hair.

I'll touch my knees,
　　my neck, my nose,
Then I'll dip down
　　and touch my toes.

Here is baby's tousled head
　　(closed fist)
She nods and nods
　　(bend fist back and forth)
Let's put her to bed.
　　(bend other arm, tuck fist into bent elbow)

Ventre de son

(Touch in order as you chant: baby's navel, midriff, chest, throat, chin, mouth,
nose, both cheeks in turn, both eyes in turn, both eyebrows in turn.)

Ventre de son,
Estomac de plomb,
Gorge de pigeon,
Menton fourchu,
Bouche d'argent,
Nez cancan,
Joue bouillie,
Joue rôtie,
P'tit oeil,
Gros oeil,
Sourcillon,
Sourcillette.

(Finish by tapping baby's forehead and saying:)

Pan, pan pan!
Cogne la caboche.

Windshield wiper, windshield wiper
What do you do all day?
Slip-slap, slip-slap,
I wipe the rain away.

(Move your hands and then baby's hands from side to side.)

~

I hold my fingers like a fish
And wave them as I go
Through the water with a swish
So gaily to and fro.

(Sing while washing baby's hands.)

~

Here is my book, I can open it wide
  (Palms of hands together, then apart)
To show the pictures that are inside.
Here is my ball so big and round
  (Make a ball with your fingers)
That I toss in the air, or roll on the ground.
  (pretend to toss up or to roll)
Here is my umbrella that keeps me dry
  (hold hand above your head, fingers spread)
When rain drops fall from the cloudy sky.
And here is my pussy, just hear her purr
When I gently stroke her soft warm fur.
  (Left hand is stroked by right hand)

~

The little train ran up the track,
It went toot, toot,
And then came back.

The other train went up the track,
It went toot, toot,
And then came back.

(Hand runs up one arm of baby and then the other.)

This little bird flaps its wings,
Flaps its wings, flaps its wings,
This little bird flaps its wings
And flies away in the morning!

(Hold up your hands with palms towards you; cross one wrist over the other and link thumbs, keeping fingers together. Move your fingers on the word "flaps," then make hands "fly away.")

Leg Rhymes

For Daddy

Leg over leg as the dog went to Dover.
When he came to a stile, "jump" he went over.

(Cross your knees and sit the baby on your ankle, holding her hands. Bounce her to the rhyme. On "jump," give her a big swing as you uncross your knees. Or sit baby on your knees with her back to you and bounce her up and down. At "jump," open your knees and let her slip down.)

Sur le dos d'une petite souris

Je partis de Lévis, sur le dos d'un p'tit' souris.
J'arrivai à Nicolet, sur le dos d'un' p'tit' belette.
A Sorel, à Sorel, sur le dos d'un' sauterelle.
A Montréal, à Montréal, sur le dos d'un orignal.
A Berthier, à Berthier, sur le dos d'un' araignée.
A Portneuf, à Portneuf, sur le dos rond d'un gros boeuf.
Je me rends à Québec, c'est pour avoir un beau bec.

(Sit with crossed legs and holding baby by the hands, balance her on your foot; make your foot jump as you accent each phrase.)

7/ From Eighteen Months to Two Years

The baby new to earth and sky,
*   What time its tender palm is pressed*
*   Against the circle of the breast,*
Has never thought that "This is I";

But as he grows he gathers much,
*   And learns the use of "I" and "me,"*
*   And finds "I am not what I see,*
And other than the things I touch."

Alfred, Lord Tennyson
(from "In Memoriam")

Our one-and-a-half-year-old keeps herself and you on the go from morning to night. She wants to explore everything, look at everything, listen to everything. Although she does not actually know how to play with other toddlers, she is interested in them and likes to have them around, and she is very proud of all the things she can do. She can open doors, go up and down stairs, kick and throw a ball, build four bricks or more, pour water from one cup to another, and feed herself quite well — if she feels like it. As her abilities grow, so does her nuisance value, and this is a period when everyone looking after her needs patience and endurance.

Increasingly vocal, she can probably say at least twelve words clearly — some in combination, is much more aware of herself as a distinct person, and has learned to indicate most of the parts of her body. She likes to listen to stories, and realizes that everything has a sound and a name; she also likes to play with sounds and words, often repeating one word over and over. Rhythmical speech play is still important, and you can now be a little more sophisticated. Instead of

72

merely imitating her, clap and chant some easy nonsense rhymes to introduce a variety of vowels and consonants:

> Cat, bat, hat, rat, all sitting on a mat
> Eny, meny, miny, mo, catcha baby by the toe
> Pitter patter, pitter patter, listen to the rain
> Fee, fi, fo, fum, Big giant I come
> Hicklety, picklety poppety pet, splash in the puddles and get all wet
> Blowing blowing windy weather ooOOoo ooOOoo ooOOoo
> (make your voice go up and down)

She will clap with you as you chant and may attempt to make some of these sounds.

Your toddler can now jump as well as trot and run, and you can tap out a variety of rhythms for her on a drum or table. When she tries to play these rhythms herself, you can accompany her on another instrument or sing or move to her playing. She will enjoy this because she loves company in any new activity. Vigorous outdoor play is essential to use up her energy, so many of the outdoor songs found in the two-year-old section can be tried now.

Unfortunately the advances of this period are accompanied by some frustrations. Although there are many things that she wants to do, there are also many things that, although necessary, she does not want to do. Music can be used to win her co-operation or distract her from an unwanted activity. With the right singing game you can coax her out of the bath, into bed, into her clothes, to come when you want her, and to eat her food. On the whole, though, eating is a serious business and it is better not to play games with food. Stories or poems or an occasional song may help at feeding time if baby is overtired or not feeling well, but these distractions should be used mainly to assure her that she has your attention. The songs included in this book that refer to food are not necessarily ones to sing when there are eating problems.

Obviously you cannot use music all the time as a distraction, nor should you, for the toddler needs to learn what is expected of her; but you must recognize that at this age she lives in the immediate present and has little concept of past or future. What is happening to her at this moment is of major importance, even though it may not seem of much importance to you. She is now very much aware that some things belong to her, and other things belong to other people; her food, her socks, her toys — all matter intensely to her. This new feeling of possession requires adjustment on your part and on hers.

If singing can help get things done faster, more easily, and with less friction, it is a boon. Songs that contribute to the toddler's sense of order and security — "This is the way we put on our coat," "One two buckle my shoe," "Mary wears red socks," etc. — not only help her (and you) through an activity but also teach her to listen; and when she listens, she is learning to concentrate, an important step in her intellectual development.

Because of her tremendous output of energy, our toddler needs a short rest during the day, and this is a good time to play some music for her, either on the record player or on an instrument. She may not sleep, but she will be resting and relaxing. The relaxing aspect of music is recognized by farmers, who play music in the dairy because their cows yield more milk as a result. Supermarkets pipe in music because they know it relaxes their customers, who then linger and buy more. Dentists value music because it has a comforting effect on their patients. So you can be sure that music can help soothe your child. Commercially piped music, however, is not the answer for the baby; it is too bland and often musically meaningless. The solution is in your own home — in your voice, your records, and your selection of radio music.

The music you play at these times not only has an immediate, short-lived effect, but also it will be added to the store of music which she will remember, either consciously or subconsciously. A friend of mine told me that when he was eighteen months old he underwent a serious operation and was in pain for some considerable time afterwards. When nothing seemed to soothe him, his mother, who was a good musician, played to him so that he was able to forget the pain and go to sleep. Today, he enjoys music and also turns to it as a source of strength and refreshment when he is tired or depressed.

When you play to your child or put on a record, show her the music or record jacket first and tell her the name of the music so that she feels that it is specially for her. If she likes what is played, she will ask for it another time, and her musical knowledge will have grown.

She is still only vaguely aware of the concepts of "big and little," "high and low," variations in shapes, and differences in colours, and this developing awareness can be strengthened through a musical approach.

One way to show contrasts is to tell the story of the three bears, emphasizing that Papa Bear is big and has a low voice, Mama Bear is middle-sized and has a middle-sized voice, and Baby Bear is tiny and has a little, high voice. The voices can be sung or played on an instrument — low, middle, high. As she listens, moves, and sings to the music, her feeling for big, middle-sized, and tiny will be intensified, as will her understanding of low, middle, and high pitch. Another song you could sing for her could describe a small sailboat, a fat tug, and a big ferry; she can stretch out her arms for the sails, run around chugging like a tug, and she may want to build the big boat with chairs. Any three subjects will do equally well as long as they are familiar to her: a car, a bus, a train; a little ball, a bigger ball, a huge balloon.

Here is a rhyme which takes her a step farther in the big and little concept and also introduces numbers: One is a giant who stamps her feet,/ Two is a fairy light and neat,/ Three is a mouse who is oh so small,/ Four is a great big bouncing ball.

Another musical way to help the baby recognize both shape and colour is to cut out three paper shapes in different colours: a round red one, a blue triangle, and a yellow oblong. Then give her a drum and while she is playing it show her the round red paper; next, give her a small easy-to-hold triangle and show her the blue triangular paper; and finally, match a chime bar with the yellow rectangle. After she has enjoyed playing with each of the three instruments, see if she can play the one that matches the coloured paper you hold up, then reverse the process by playing each instrument yourself and encouraging the toddler to pick up the matching piece of paper. This game may be a little advanced for the eighteen to twenty-two-month old, but it is certainly possible to introduce to the two-year-old. All such games help the baby appreciate size, shape, colour, and sound. Because they are more fun when played with two or three other children, they help in the socializing process.

For some time now you have been singing her name to the sol-fa sounds: soh-me. If you have a piano or if she has some chime bars, you have been letting her find top and bottom doh and soh and me. Because lah comes into so many easy nursery rhymes you very likely have introduced it too. Now that she is aware of colours, you may stick coloured paper on her chime bars, or on the piano keys, or even on a group of blocks. The colours will then represent the sounds being sung. You can sing the notes and let the baby find them, and then ask her to tell you their colour; or you can name the colour and let her sing the correct sound. A melody can be written on a blackboard or large sheet of paper using coloured notes so that when you sing it, she can see as well as hear how the tune moves along the staff.

Here is a chart of associated notes and colours used by Mary Helen Richards at her Institute in Portola Valley, California, which you will find useful.

Black	Green	Blue	Orange	Red	Yellow	Brown
d	r	m	f	s	l	t

The tonic sol-fa hand signs invented by John Curwen in 1816, and popularized in recent years by Zoltán Kodály, are helpful because the toddler not only hears but also sees and can make these signs, thus involving the whole child in learning about pitch. The important pitch levels involve soh, me, doh and lah, but ray can also be introduced, as it completes the five-note (pentatonic) scale, which is used for so many of the early folk and nursery rhyme melodies.

Here are the hand signs that you are most likely to use, and a line of a song "Pitter Patter" to illustrate them.

Sol-fa Hands Signs

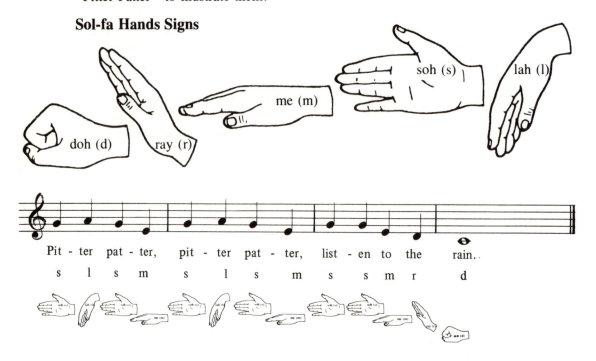

When keeping time, you may find it helpful to sing the names of the musical notes that Curwen introduced, for they accurately represent the time value of each note. He used French, though Kodály changed the sounds of some of them to suit the Hungarian language. Here are the basic ones and part of the song "Bye Baby Bunting" to illustrate their use. Your toddler will be able to clap and sing easy rhythmic patterns by using them.

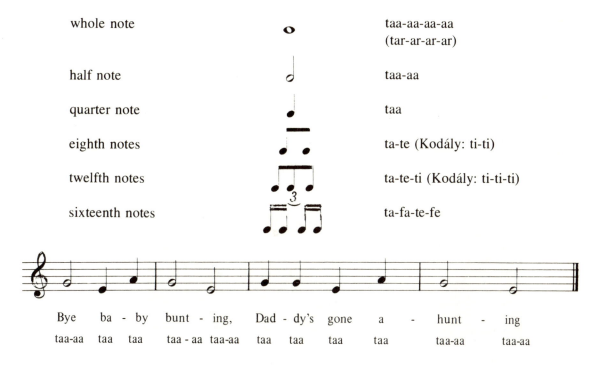

whole note	taa-aa-aa-aa (tar-ar-ar-ar)
half note	taa-aa
quarter note	taa
eighth notes	ta-te (Kodály: ti-ti)
twelfth notes	ta-te-ti (Kodály: ti-ti-ti)
sixteenth notes	ta-fa-te-fe

Bye   ba - by   bunt - ing,   Dad - dy's   gone   a   -   hunt - ing
taa-aa taa taa taa - aa taa-aa taa taa taa taa taa-aa taa-aa

This is a marvellous age for trying out all kinds of home-made instruments, and again this is an occupation which lends itself to a group of toddlers. Given instruments of different shapes, sizes, and colours that produce different sounds they will swap the instruments constantly, choosing on the basis of size, shape, colour or sound, and this is not only fun but helps to teach them discrimination.

Examples of Galloping Rhythm

Charlie Is My Darling

Scottish

Pop Goes the Weasel

Nursery Rhyme

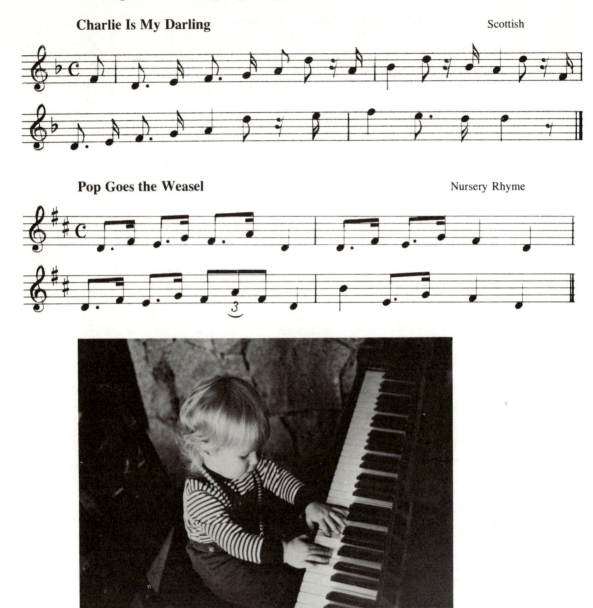

Example of Skipping Rhythm

Girls and Boys Come Out to Play   English

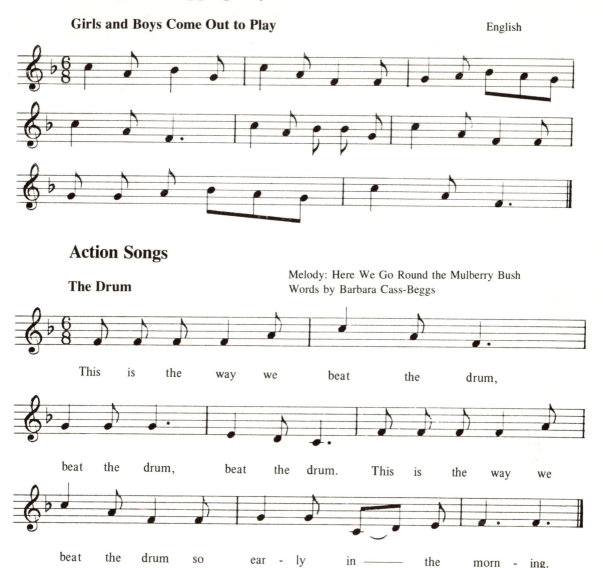

Action Songs

The Drum

Melody: Here We Go Round the Mulberry Bush
Words by Barbara Cass-Beggs

This is the way we beat the drum,

beat the drum, beat the drum. This is the way we

beat the drum so ear - ly in —— the morn - ing.

Use other instruments in turn.

German Folk Melody
Words adapted by Barbara Cass-Beggs

The Band

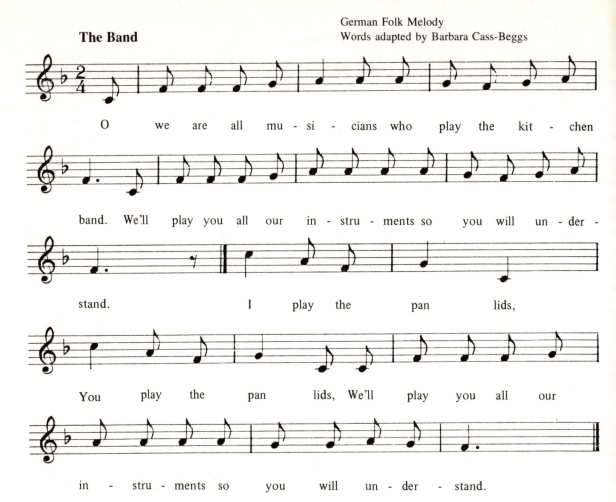

O we are all mu-si-cians who play the kit-chen

band. We'll play you all our in-stru-ments so you will un-der-

stand. I play the pan lids,

You play the pan lids, We'll play you all our

in-stru-ments so you will un-der-stand.

To be used with a group of children. Everyone plays the first section together, then one child plays solo, a different instrument being played each time. Percussion instruments can be used in place of kitchen pots and pans.

Mary Wears a Red Dress

Melody: London Bridge Is Falling Down
Words suggested by Ruth Crawford Seeger

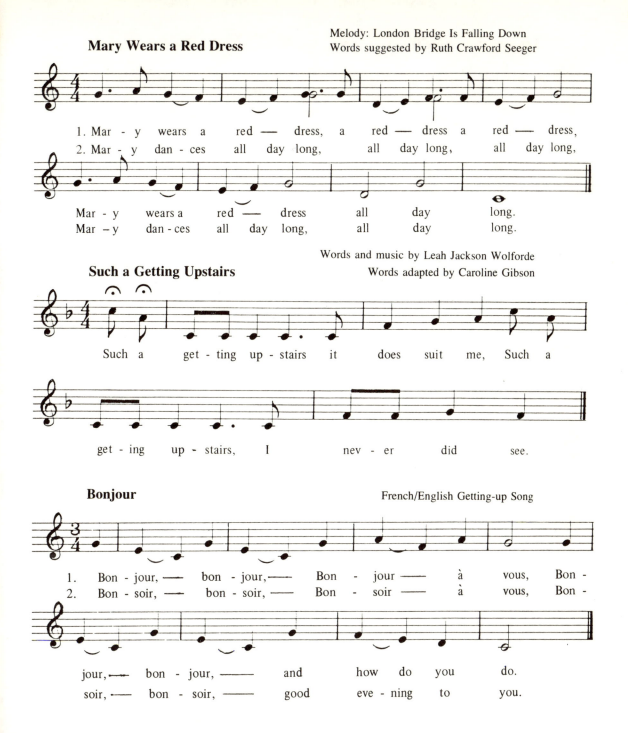

1. Mar - y wears a red — dress, a red — dress a red — dress,
2. Mar - y dan - ces all day long, all day long, all day long,

Mar - y wears a red — dress all day long.
Mar - y dan - ces all day long, all day long.

Such a Getting Upstairs

Words and music by Leah Jackson Wolforde
Words adapted by Caroline Gibson

Such a get - ting up - stairs it does suit me, Such a

get - ing up - stairs, I nev - er did see.

Bonjour

French/English Getting-up Song

1. Bon - jour, — bon - jour, — Bon - jour — à vous, Bon -
2. Bon - soir, — bon - soir, — Bon - soir — à vous, Bon -

jour, — bon - jour, — and how do you do.
soir, — bon - soir, — good eve - ning to you.

Les menottes sautent   French Nursery Song

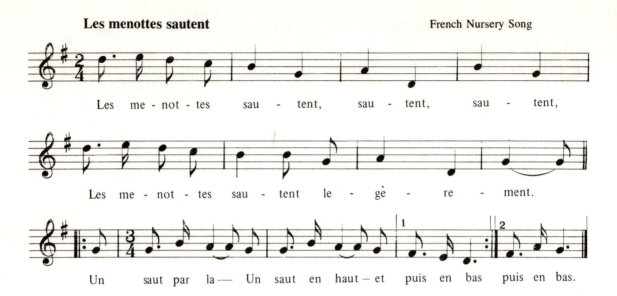

Les me - not - tes sau - tent, sau - tent, sau - tent,

Les me - not - tes sau - tent le - gè - re - ment.

Un saut par la— Un saut en haut — et puis en bas puis en bas.

Wave baby's arms over her head, then to one side and the oppostie side, up high and down low; or accompany the song with bells or rattles.

Tout la haut   Sung to author by Evy Paraskevopoulos

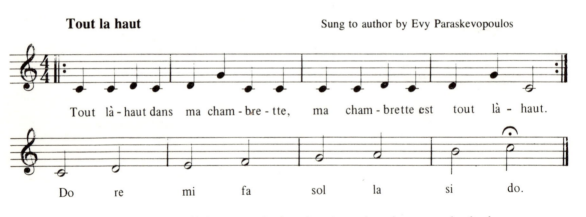

Tout là - haut dans ma cham - bre - tte, ma cham - brette est tout là - haut.

Do re mi fa sol la si do.

Move baby's arms as if she were playing the piano, keeping a steady rhythm.

Allons nous promener

Traditional Nursery chant

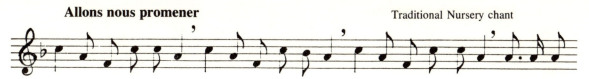

Al - lons nous pro - me-ner Par les champs par les près, Al - lons nous pro-me-ner hors de bois.

Hold baby's hands. At "hors de bois," turn her around.

Violette

French Number Rhyme

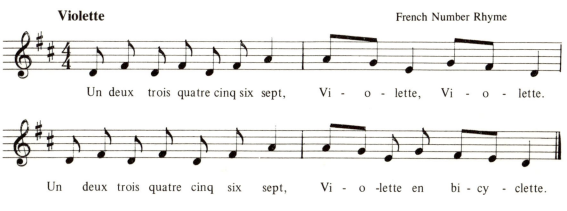

Un deux trois quatre cinq six sept, Vi - o - lette, Vi - o - lette.

Un deux trois quatre cinq six sept, Vi - o -lette en bi - cy - clette.

Move baby's legs as if she were bicycling.

Singing Games

Ring Around a Rosy

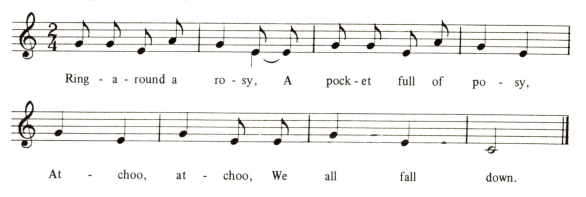

Ring - a - round a ro - sy, A pock - et full of po - sy,

At - choo, at - choo, We all fall down.

2. Cows are in the meadow,
   Lying fast asleep.
   Atchoo, atchoo, we all jump up.

84

Sally Go Round the Sun

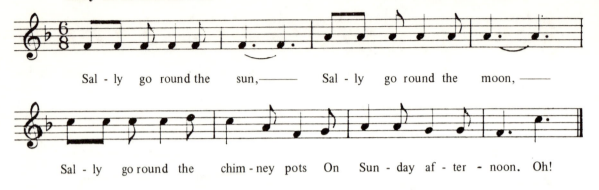

Sal - ly go round the sun,—— Sal - ly go round the moon, ——

Sal - ly go round the chim - ney pots On Sun - day af - ter - noon. Oh!

Dance in a circle and reverse on ''Oh!''

When the Ducks Get Up

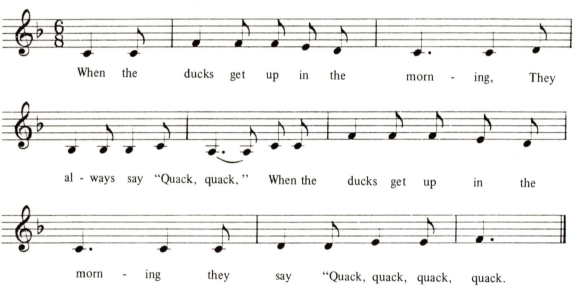

When the ducks get up in the morn - ing, They

al - ways say "Quack, quack," When the ducks get up in the

morn - ing they say "Quack, quack, quack, quack.

Suggest other animals and their sounds.

Hot Cross Buns English Nursery Rhyme

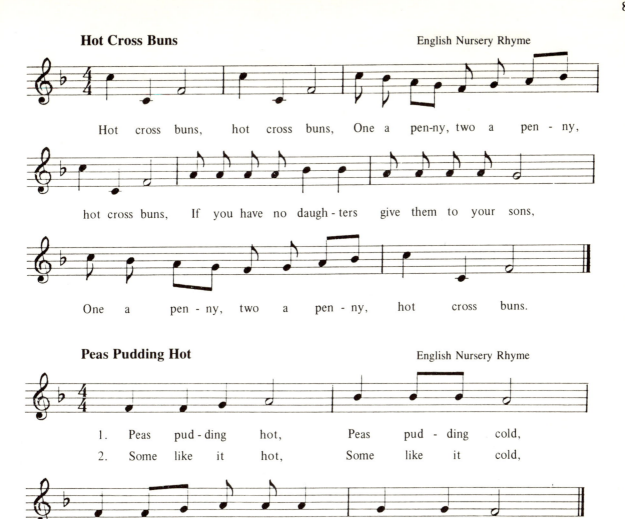

Hot cross buns, hot cross buns, One a pen-ny, two a pen - ny,

hot cross buns, If you have no daugh-ters give them to your sons,

One a pen - ny, two a pen - ny, hot cross buns.

Peas Pudding Hot English Nursery Rhyme

1. Peas pud - ding hot, Peas pud - ding cold,
2. Some like it hot, Some like it cold,

Peas pud - ding in the pot, Nine days old.
Some like it in the pot, Nine days old.

Dressing Songs

This Is the Way

Melody: Traditional
Words suggested by Ruth Crawford Seeger

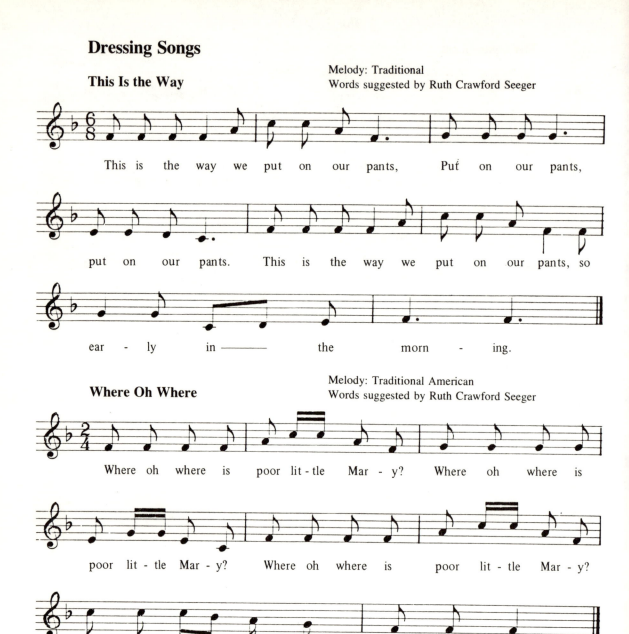

This is the way we put on our pants, Put on our pants,

put on our pants. This is the way we put on our pants, so

ear - ly in —— the morn - ing.

Where Oh Where

Melody: Traditional American
Words suggested by Ruth Crawford Seeger

Where oh where is poor lit - tle Mar - y? Where oh where is

poor lit - tle Mar - y? Where oh where is poor lit - tle Mar - y?

Way down yon - der in a tight green shirt.

A song to be sung when you have difficulty getting clothing over baby's head.

This melody can also be used to play a hiding game, using these words:

1. Where oh where is our little Mary? (repeat twice)
   We can't find her anywhere.

2. Oh, hurray, I can hear her coming (repeat twice)
   Running (crawling, walking) as fast as she can run (crawl, walk).

One Button

English Number Rhyme

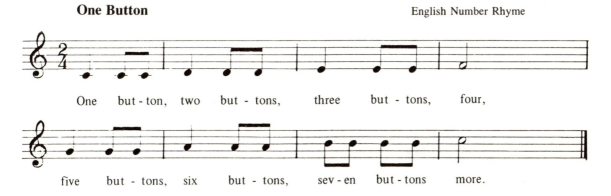

One but-ton, two but-tons, three but-tons, four, five but-tons, six but-tons, sev-en but-tons more.

Sing up the scale when buttoning baby's coat or sweater, down when unbuttoning her clothing.

One, Two, Buckle My Shoe

English Number Rhyme
Music by Barbara Cass-Beggs

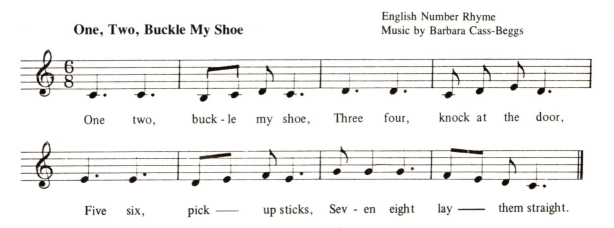

One two, buck-le my shoe, Three four, knock at the door, Five six, pick — up sticks, Sev-en eight lay — them straight.

Action Rhymes

A little ball,
A bigger ball
A great big ball I see.
   (shape hands to make a ball)
Now let us count
The balls we've made,
One, two, three.
       ~

Choo, choo, choo, choo . . .
   (rub palms together in a circular motion to make a noise, slowly at first,
   then gradually increasing speed)
Too-too, too-too, too-too . . .
   (keep hands rubbing fast as you call "too-too")
Choo-choo, choo-choo, choo-choo . . .
   (rub hands gradually more slowly)
Ding-dong, ding-dong, ding-dong.
   (when you reach the last "ding-dong," stop altogether)
       ~

Five little birds without any home,
   (raise the fingers and thumb of the right hand)
Five little trees in a row.
   (raise right hand high over your head)
Come build your nests in our branches tall
   (cup left hand for a nest, place right hand fingers in it)
We'll rock you to and fro.
   (rock both hands)
       ~

Five little kittens
All black and white
Sleeping very soundly
All through the night.
   (the hand is made into a fist for this verse)
Meow, meow, meow, meow, meow
It's time to get up now.
   (Raise a different finger for each "meow")

Up in the sky the little birds fly
    (flutter outstretched hands)
Down in their nests the little birds rest.
    (lower hands)
With a wing on the left and a wing on the right,
    (wave left hand, then right hand)
The dear little birdies sleep all night.
    (fold hands under cheek)

What can I do with both my hands,
What can I do with both my hands,
What can I do with both my hands,
Early in the morning?

Give a little clap and shake them all over
(repeat 3 times)
Early in the morning.

What can I do with both my feet
(repeat 3 times)
Early in the morning?

Give a little clap and shake them all over, etc.

What can I do with all my body, etc.
Give a little clap and shake it all over, etc.
(clap hands and feet)

(This can be sung to the tune of "What Shall We Do With the Drunken Sailor")

8 / The Two-Year Old

And when our baby stirs and struggles to be born
It compels humility: what we began
Is now its own.

Anne Ridler
(from "Nine Bright Shiners")

By the time your toddler is two she is able to do more for herself, and life gradually becomes easier. Although there are still frustrations, this is a fascinating period because she can now play with other children, and can take part in more musical activities.

She has much more control over her actions and tries not to spill or grab. Naturally, there are lapses, but she is aware of them and will be sorry for them — particularly if her lapses were deliberate and she has got what she wanted. She is beginning to have an idea of time: she can understand when you say "soon," "later," or "in a minute" — and this certainly helps. What she wants she still wants now, but it is possible to modify "now" into "just a minute," and if you keep your part of the bargain all should go well.

Her speech is more fluent and interesting. She may say up to twenty clear words, and some children have a larger vocabulary by this age. Nouns and adjectives are being used grammatically, and she can put together some simple phrases and sentences. She understands anything you say, and if she is particularly interested in words, she may ask you what a word means. You can now hear in her speech the distinct sounds of "t," "d," "n," "k," and "ng," and within the next six months, or sooner, she will establish her identity by saying "I." (I always remember my older daughter's first sentence at this age, when she came into the room wearing one of my hats and announced proudly, "Here I are.")

Many two-year-olds say very little, and there are those with such poor articulation that they are difficult to understand. Such children can be helped considerably by chanting and singing, preferably in a music group, for though they still like to play on their own, at this age they also enjoy being part of a group and will co-operate with other adults as well as with their mother.

This is an age when the toddler loves to help in all kinds of social activities, such as setting the table or putting away toys. In a music group, taking out and putting away instruments and books is therefore a very important part of the program.

Because the toddler loves to draw she can be invited to draw a picture about what the music tells her, even if it is just scribble. Some children who are advanced for their age will produce an understandable picture, sometimes including musical notes.

She enjoys playing a big drum and moving to its rhythm, and can play the rhythm of her name (Mary = ♩♩) as well as other rhythmic patterns such as ♫♩ = Teddy Bear or ♫♩ = Christmas tree. Tone blocks, rattles, bells, small sturdy tambourines and rhythm sticks can all be managed and provide exciting alternatives to the drum. She loves to sing; she can repeat songs that she has heard and can make up her own songs as she plays. She can count to two digits (more if she is particularly interested in numbers) and is ready for simple number songs.

There is still a good deal of aggression in the two-year-old, but when you divert her attention, she forgets to be angry. Playing with other children and taking turns is still not easy. She will usually take her turn, as long as she always gets it, but sometimes hers stretches into several turns! Songs can help out in a number of these difficult situations. "See-Saw Marjorie Daw" and "How Do You Like to Go Up in a Swing" are excellent for taking turns on playground equipment, and "Take My Hand" or "What Shall We Do When We All Go Out" are good socializing songs for outdoor play.

Because she likes to *be* everything as well as *do* everything, "Driving in My Car," "The Train Song," and "See the Pony" are especially popular at this age. Boats and planes are fascinating to her, as are actions associated with weather, such as splashing in puddles, sliding on ice, and running in the wind. Just as you have sung lullabies to her, so she will sing them to her doll or teddy bear. And you can help her to be aware of the feelings of animals through such songs as "Sweet Pussy, Soft Pussy," or "I Love Little Pussy."

Do not worry if she does not sing in tune. In singing, as in speech, children vary considerably; some sing in tune quite early, and others take longer. Most children acquire "relative" pitch: the ability to select and sing a series of notes correctly and to continue singing them in tune. A few children have "perfect" pitch: the ability to sing and name the exact pitch of a note from its sound alone without reference to any other note. This ability, inherited or acquired only before the age of two, is a fascinating subject, but somewhat technical. There are also children who grow up unable to distinguish or reproduce sounds of different pitch; they are described as "tone deaf" (a misleading term, since they are not deaf) or "monotones." The genuine monotone is rare. So is the child with perfect pitch, which though it seems a very wonderful acquisition has its drawbacks and is not synonymous with musical ability. Experience shows that the child from a musical family invariably enjoys music and will sing more easily in tune, and usually accomplishes more musically than a child from a non-musical family.

You can help your toddler to sing in tune by singing her songs in a lower key than you would normally sing them, for research indicates that two- and three-year-olds naturally pitch a song lower (for example, B or B♭ below middle C). Be sure that she hears the first, or starting, note of a piece correctly (if not, she may become confused and be thrown off pitch), and do not sing too fast. You have seen adults walking along with their two-year-old running to keep up with them; it is the same with singing. The pace and words must be slow enough for the toddler to keep up with the music. If she cannot keep up, she will not enjoy singing, and if she does not enjoy it, she will not learn.

When your toddler can sing with more or less correct rhythm and pitch, and with some feeling for loudness or softness and quickness or slowness, she is exercising auditory discrimination, an important factor in her development and one allied with reading ability and verbal skills. Toddlers have been tested for their "listening" ability, and though more needs to be done in this area, enough tests have been given to show that listening discrimination depends on the variety of sounds, including music, they hear and how these sounds are introduced, particularly the avoidance of too much noise and repetition. This explains why children from economically poor families who often grow up in an over-crowded and noisy environment and one that provides little musical variety usually have reading problems and need help in acquiring verbal skills.

92

Not only does music help a toddler's ability to discriminate and adjust socially, but it also contributes to her sense of security. Today, when families move frequently, a familiar house, tree, garden, or school will be left behind, but the family music can go along; the same reassuring sounds can be recreated wherever the family is. The crib springs will still squeak, the pots and pans will still make lovely clashing sounds, and mother's lullaby is still the same. Many familiar songs will be sung in the new pre-school or day care centre, too. In fact, moving is a good time for the family to make up new songs:

One, two, what shall we do?
Unpack the furniture, find the lost shoe,
Find baby's bottle, have something to eat,
Now we are ready for bath time and sleep.

Car travelling can be very boring for the active toddler, but poems and nursery rhymes or even just making noises can help pass the time, as long as the noises are not so loud that they upset the driver. Singing is perhaps best, for everyone can join in, and mother or father can make the music more interesting by trying to harmonize. Even the wrong notes can be fun, and if your children know that they are wrong, you can be pleased that they can tell the difference. Older children can join in with recorders or harmonicas, and the two-year-old need not be left out, for a piece of tissue paper over a comb makes a happy sound. So does a simple whistle, though too much repetition of one or possibly two notes can be hard on the ears! When the young ones begin to get sleepy, a lullaby is always in order, and the journey will be over before you know it.

When the toddler is being cared for by someone other than her mother, or is attending a day care centre, however good the environment may be, it will be a tiring, and for some a difficult, experience. Music not only provides a link with home, but can also offer the child a much needed energy release, followed by an equally necessary rest and relaxation period. Toddlers frequently become emotionally tense and frustrated, and a session of drum playing, stamping, and pretending to be different things help to play out some of these emotions. The shy child who wants to play with others but finds it difficult can be helped to feel part of the group when everyone is singing or taking part in a singing game. Music can also provide individual attention, which every two-year-old still needs.

A period of music each day is good, but it is better still if music can be included in every part of the daily routine. One of the most trying times of day for two-year-olds is the waking period after rest. When they are still sleepy, they are apt to be cross, and do not want to do anything until they have had a snack. One group care centre solved this problem by letting the children who were up first put on records of their own choosing. As the others awoke, they gathered around the record player to listen, and this seemed to fill the gap between sleeping and waking. This technique could be tried at home, too.

Although most books on child care designate this age as "the terrible twos," I have not found it to be so as far as music is concerned. It may be that because two-year-olds can do more than is usually expected of them, they become frustrated and "terrible" if not challenged. I have been amazed at what the twos can do musically when they are concentrating, and though they cannot concentrate for long stretches, their attention span is considerable if you move fairly quickly from one aspect of the same subject to another.

The conditions under which a child's body best develops are given in Charles Corbin's *A Text Book of Motor Development*, and as many of these are the same conditions under which a baby's musical ability will develop, I have included some of them here:

Learning must be a happy experience.
There must be a free, flexible learning environment.
The baby's abilities and interests must set the pace.
Adequate living and play area are necessary.
Too much teaching of details must be avoided.
Vigorous activity must be alternated with less vigorous activity.
There must be no pressure to try things that are too difficult for the child.
Play must be recognized as the best way to achieve learning.
Behaviour must not be strictly channeled.
Every baby must have encouragement and support.
Children are so different that there must be no attempt to classify their progress.

In these two years your infant has *lived* through her experiences rather than *thought* about them. Because unconscious absorbtion through action aids a child's growing intelligence, she needs a stimulating environment which she can explore during the sensitive period of birth to two years. Educator Maria Montessori describes the normal infant as one who has a sense of order; a desire to work (any activity that absorbs the child's whole personality); a profound, spontaneous concentration; an appreciation of reality; an enjoyment of silence; and a sense of independence, initiative, and joy. No wonder that parents feel they have a big responsibility. I am reminded of a friend who was adopting a baby boy. Having stated her credentials and having been given the information about the baby, she said: "Well, it isn't a question of whether he is good enough for us; it is a question of whether *we* are good enough for him!"

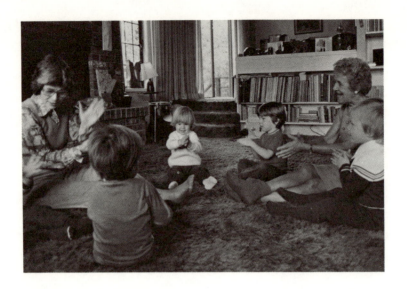

Outdoor Songs

Take My Hand

Words and music by Barbara Cass-Beggs

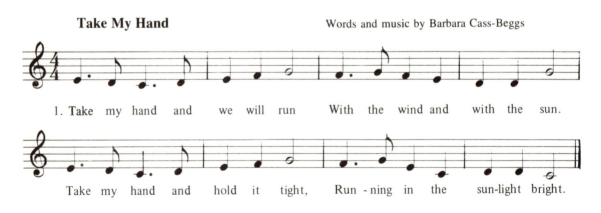

1. Take my hand and we will run With the wind and with the sun.

Take my hand and hold it tight, Run-ning in the sun-light bright.

2. Take my mitten, in the snow,
   Dodging snowflakes we will go.
   Take my mitt and hold it tight
   As we watch the snow in flight.

3. Take my hand as home we go,
   Running, walking, not too slow.
   Take my hand and you will see
   Just how happy we can be.

It's Blowing

Words and music by Barbara Cass-Beggs

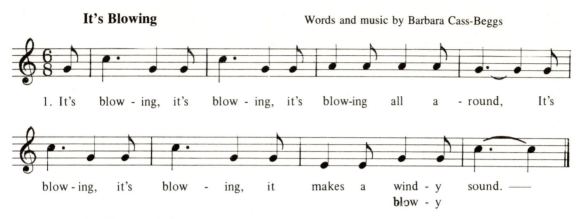

1. It's blow-ing, it's blow-ing, it's blow-ing all a - round, It's
blow-ing, it's blow - ing, it makes a wind - y sound. ——
blow - y

2. It's snowing, etc.
   It does not make a sound.

3. It's raining, etc.
   It's dropping on the ground.
   (It patters)

I Hear Thunder

Melody: Traditional French (Frère Jacques)

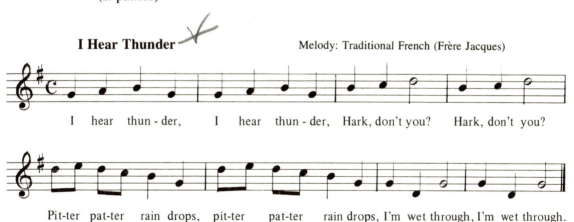

I hear thun-der, I hear thun-der, Hark, don't you? Hark, don't you?

Pit-ter pat-ter rain drops, pit-ter pat-ter rain drops, I'm wet through, I'm wet through.

If indoors, stomp or pound on the floor to make thunder; put your hand to your
ear for "Hark, don't you?"; make raindrops by wriggling your fingers, and hug
yourself for "I'm wet through."

Riding In My Car

Words and music by Woody Guthrie

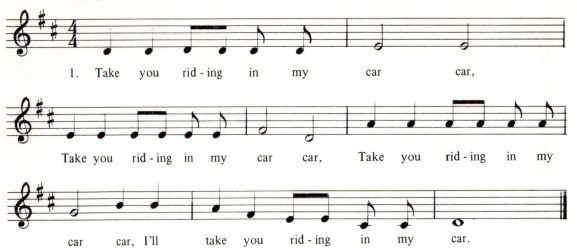

1. Take you rid-ing in my car car,
Take you rid-ing in my car car, Take you rid-ing in my
car car, I'll take you rid-ing in my car.

2. Click-a-clack open up the door, girls,
Click-a-clack open up the door, boys,
Front door, back door, clickety clack,
Take you riding in my car.

3. Climb climb rattle on the front seat
Spree, spraddle on the back seat,
Turn the key, start the engine,
I'll take you riding in my car.

4. The engine it goes brrm brrm,
(repeat 3 times)
Take you riding in my car.

5. Brrm-brrm chrrka-chrrka, brrm-brrm, (repeat 3 times)
We've been riding in my car.

6. Grownups nod as we go by,
Children laugh as we go by,
They all wave as we go by,
Riding in my car.

7. I'm gonna let you blow the horn,
I'm gonna let you blow the horn,
Beep, beep, beep, beep —
Riding in my car.

8. Now I'm gonna drive you home again (repeat 3 times)
Riding in my car.

(Repeat verses 4 and 5 between other verses.)

Bunny (Easter Song)

German Folk Melody
Words by Barbara Cass-Beggs

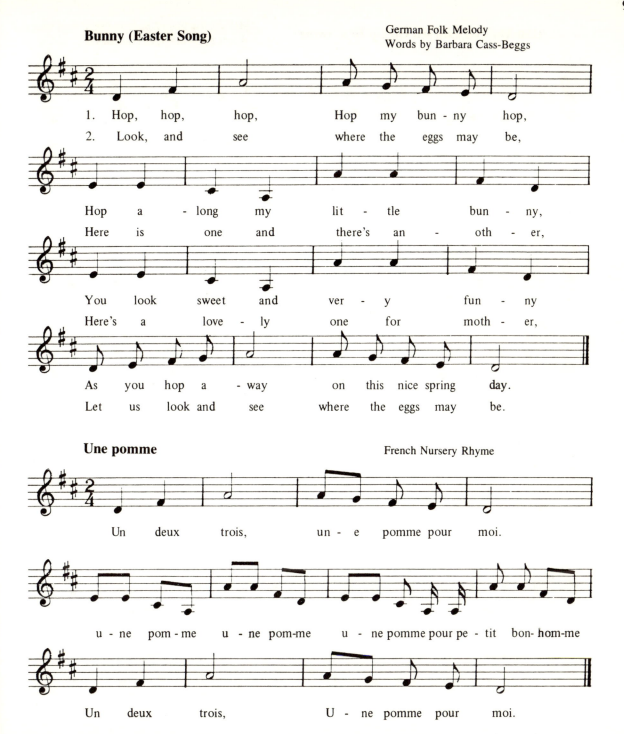

1. Hop, hop, hop, Hop my bun-ny hop,
2. Look, and see where the eggs may be,

Hop a - long my lit - tle bun - ny,
Here is one and there's an - oth - er,

You look sweet and ver - y fun - ny
Here's a love - ly one for moth - er,

As you hop a - way on this nice spring **day.**
Let us look and see where the eggs may be.

Une pomme

French Nursery Rhyme

Un deux trois, un - e pomme pour moi.

u - ne pom - me u - ne pom-me u - ne pomme pour pe - tit bon- hom-me

Un deux trois, U - ne pomme pour moi.

How Do You Like To Go Up In a Swing

Melody: Traditional Scottish (Skye Boat Song)
Words by Robert Louis Stevenson

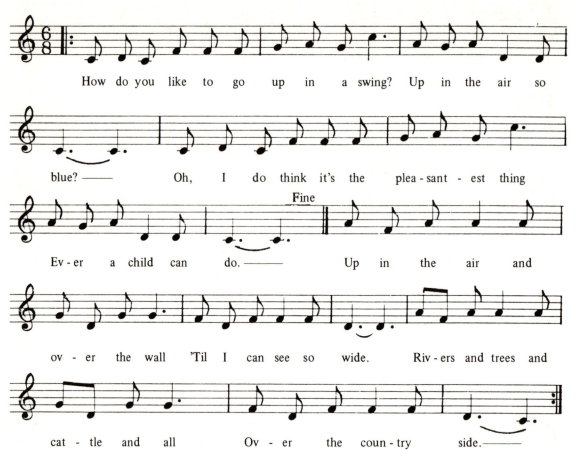

How do you like to go up in a swing? Up in the air so

blue? —— Oh, I do think it's the plea-sant-est thing

Fine

Ev-er a child can do. —— Up in the air and

ov-er the wall 'Til I can see so wide. Riv-ers and trees and

cat-tle and all Ov-er the coun-try side.——

Papillons volez

French Nursery Rhyme

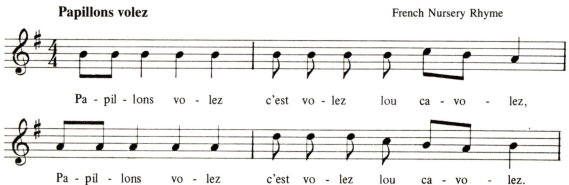

Pa-pil-lons vo-lez c'est vo-lez lou ca-vo-lez,

Pa-pil-lons vo-lez c'est vo-lez lou ca-vo-lez.

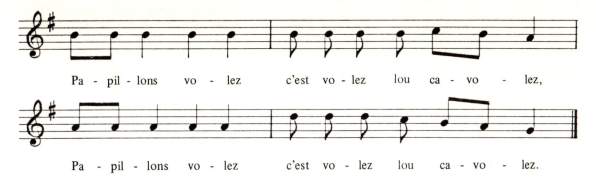

Pa - pil - lons   vo - lez   c'est vo - lez lou ca - vo - lez,

Pa - pil - lons   vo - lez   c'est vo - lez lou ca - vo - lez.

Fly around the yard like butterflies or make fluttering butterfly movements with your hands while sitting.

The Bus

Anon. Nursery Song

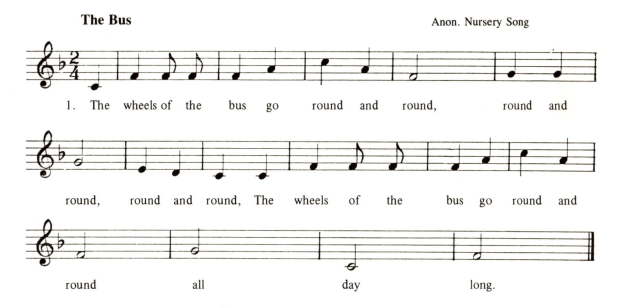

1. The wheels of the   bus   go   round and   round,   round and

round,   round and round, The   wheels of   the   bus   go round and

round   all   day   long.

2. The horn on the bus goes beep beep beep, etc.
3. The wipers of the bus go swish swish swish etc.
4. The driver of the bus says "Move back please," etc.
5. There's a sign on the road that says "Please stop here," etc.
   So we all get down.

Trains

Melody: Traditional English
Words by Barbara Cass-Beggs from an
idea by S. N. Coleman and A.G. Thorn

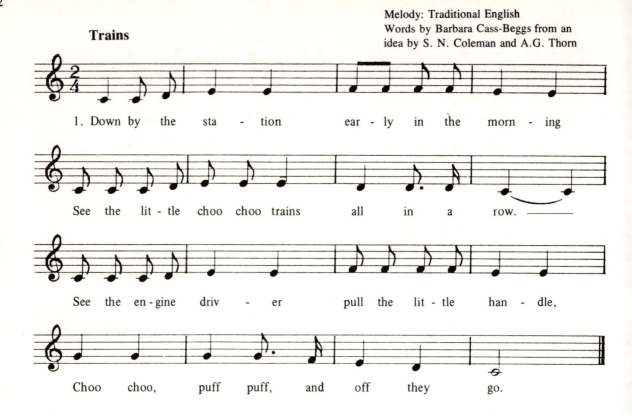

1. Down by the sta - tion ear - ly in the morn - ing

See the lit - tle choo choo trains all in a row. ———

See the en - gine driv - er pull the lit - tle han - dle,

Choo choo, puff puff, and off they go.

2. Down at the harbour early in the morning
   See the little tug boats waiting to go.
   See the tugboat captain starting up the engine,
   Chug, chug, toot toot, and off they go.

3. Early in the morning, down at the airport
   See the big jet liners all in a row.
   Propellers now are whirring and everyone is ready,
   Brr brr, boom boom, and up they go.

Big Jet Planes

Words and music by Barbara Cass-Beggs

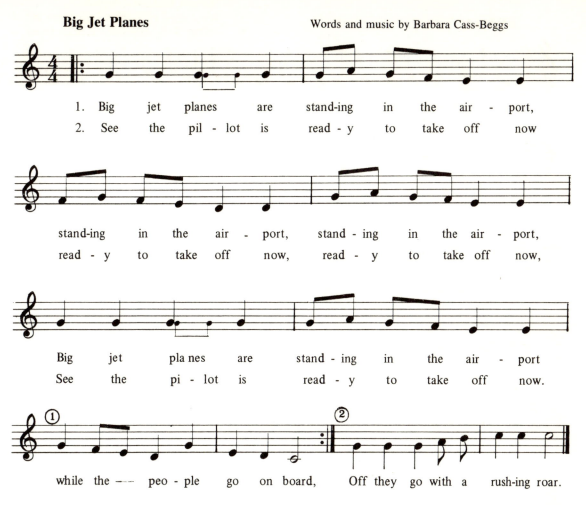

1. Big jet planes are stand-ing in the air - port,
2. See the pil - lot is read - y to take off now

stand-ing in the air - port, stand - ing in the air - port,
read - y to take off now, read - y to take off now,

Big jet pla nes are stand - ing in the air - port
See the pi - lot is read - y to take off now.

while the — peo - ple go on board, Off they go with a rush-ing roar.

3. They are flying way up in the clouds now, etc.
   We no longer see them there.

This verse can be played an octave higher, using the second ending.

I Went to Visit

Anon.

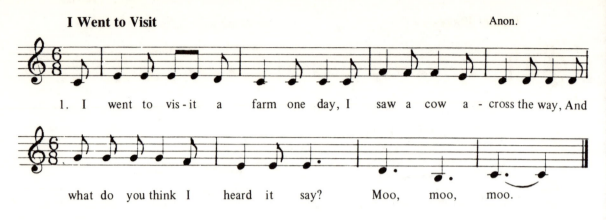

1. I went to vis-it a farm one day, I saw a cow a-cross the way, And

what do you think I heard it say? Moo, moo, moo.

Substitute a horse, a dog, a cat, a hen, etc.

2. I went to visit a town one day,
   I saw a bus across the way,
   And what do you think I heard it say?
   Brmm, brmm, brmm.

Substitute a bike (swish, swish),
a car (beep, beep or toot, toot)

Indoor Songs

Here's a Ball

Words and music by Emile Poulson

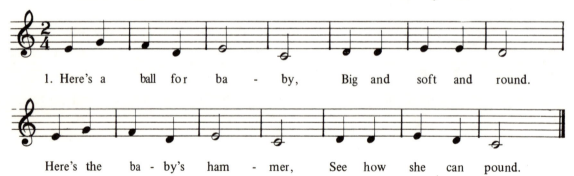

1. Here's a ball for ba - by, Big and soft and round.

Here's the ba - by's ham - mer, See how she can pound.

2. Here's the baby's music, clapping clapping so,
   Here are baby's soldiers standing in a row.
3. Here's the baby's trumpet, toot-a-toot-a-too.
   This is how our baby plays at peek-a-boo!
4. Here's the big umbrella, keeps the baby dry.
   Here's the baby's cradle, hush-a-baby-bye.

Used with permission of Stainer & Bell, Ltd., London, publishers.

Watch My Dogs

Melody: Twinkle, Twinkle Little Star
Words by Barbara Cass-Beggs
from an idea of Marion Anderson

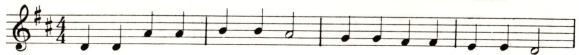

1. Watch my dogs and you will see They walk al - ways one two three.

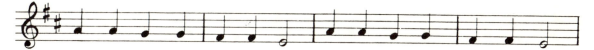

First the brown dog leads the line, Then the white with fur so fine,

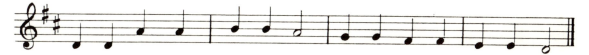

Black dog fol - lows and you'll see They walk al - ways one two three.

2. Watch my bears and you will see
   They walk always one two three.
   First the big bear pads around,
   Then the black with nose on ground.
   Brown bear follows from his tree,
   Watch them walking, one two three.

3. Watch my children, you will see
   They walk always one two three.
   First comes John to lead the line,
   Then Michelle with smile so fine.
   Susan follows and you see
   They walk always one two three.

I Love Little Pussy

English Nursery Rhyme

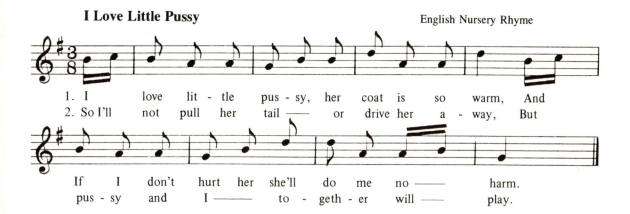

1. I love lit - tle pus - sy, her coat is so warm, And
2. So I'll not pull her tail — or drive her a - way, But

If I don't hurt her she'll do me no — harm.
pus - sy and I — to - geth - er will — play.

106

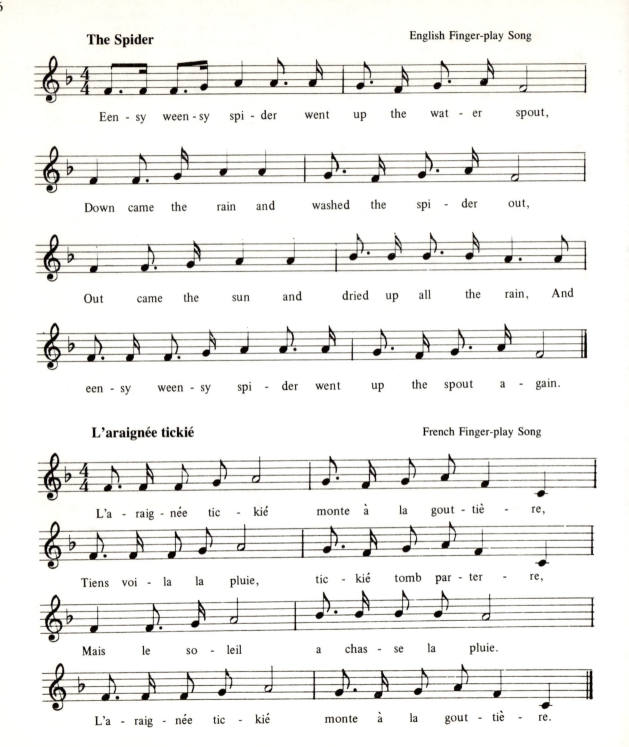

The Spider
English Finger-play Song

Een - sy ween - sy spi - der went up the wat - er spout,

Down came the rain and washed the spi - der out,

Out came the sun and dried up all the rain, And

een - sy ween - sy spi - der went up the spout a - gain.

L'araignée tickié
French Finger-play Song

L'a - raig - née tic - kié monte à la gout - tiè - re,

Tiens voi - la la pluie, tic - kié tomb par - ter - re,

Mais le so - leil a chas - se la pluie.

L'a - raig - née tic - kié monte à la gout - tiè - re.

Rain

Words and music by Barbara Cass-Beggs

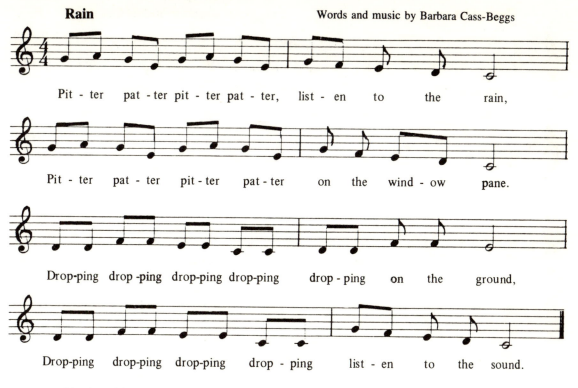

Pit - ter pat -ter pit - ter pat - ter, list - en to the rain,

Pit - ter pat - ter pit - ter pat - ter on the wind - ow pane.

Drop-ping drop -ping drop-ping drop-ping drop - ping on the ground,

Drop-ping drop-ping drop-ping drop - ping list - en to the sound.

Singing this song helps a child with his "p"s, "l"s and "r"s. The first part of the melody is easy to play on chime bars or the piano, and it is a good rhythm for rhythm sticks.

Neige neige blanche

French Nursery Song

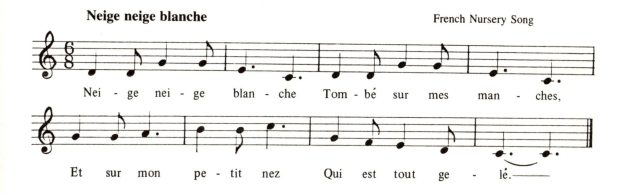

Nei - ge nei - ge blan - che Tom - bé sur mes man - ches,

Et sur mon pe - tit nez Qui est tout ge - lé.

Pussy Cat

Swiss Folk Melody
Words adapted by Barbara Cass-Beggs

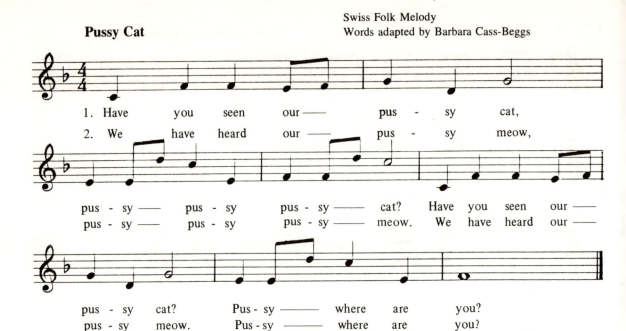

1. Have you seen our —— pus - sy cat,
2. We have heard our —— pus - sy meow,

pus - sy —— pus - sy pus - sy —— cat? Have you seen our ——
pus - sy —— pus - sy pus - sy —— meow. We have heard our ——

pus - sy cat? Pus - sy —— where are you?
pus - sy meow. Pus - sy —— where are you?

In this song-game, baby hides while you sing the first verse, then says "meow"
for the second verse, crawls to you and lets you stroke her.

Baby Jump Up

Variation on Hush-a-bye Baby
Words and music by Barbara Cass-Beggs

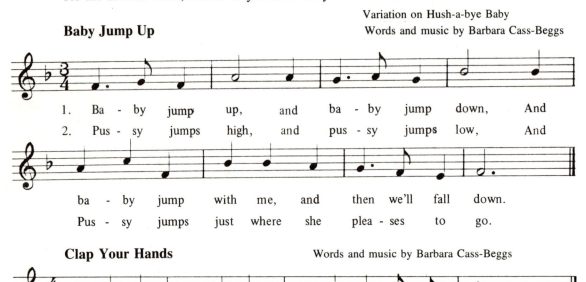

1. Ba - by jump up, and ba - by jump down, And
2. Pus - sy jumps high, and pus - sy jumps low, And

ba - by jump with me, and then we'll fall down.
Pus - sy jumps just where she plea - ses to go.

Clap Your Hands

Words and music by Barbara Cass-Beggs

Clap your hands, clap your hands, clap your hands 'til the mu - sic stops.

2. Stamp your feet, etc.　　　3. Wave your arms, etc.

Who's That

American Folk Song

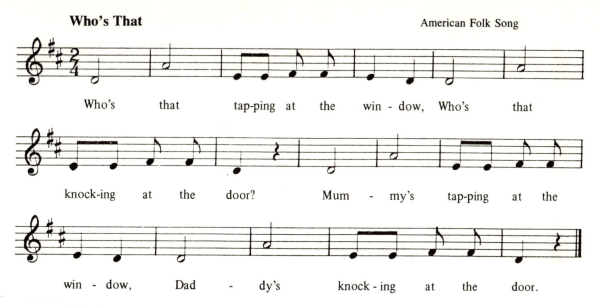

Who's that tap-ping at the win - dow, Who's that knock-ing at the door? Mum - my's tap-ping at the win - dow, Dad - dy's knock - ing at the door.

This is an excellent song for introducing loud and soft.

Reprinted by permission of the publishers from Dorothy Scarborough, ON THE TRAIL OF NEGRO FOLK-SONGS, Cambridge, Mass.: Harvard University Press, Copyright ©1925 by Harvard University Press; 1953 by Mary McDaniel Parker.

The Ice-Cream Man

Traditional English Singing Game
Words adapted by Barbara Cass-Beggs

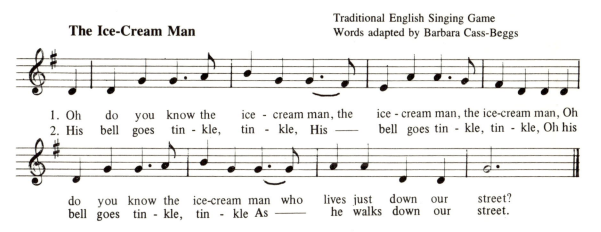

1. Oh do you know the ice - cream man, the ice - cream man, the ice-cream man, Oh do you know the ice-cream man who lives just down our street?
2. His bell goes tin - kle, tin - kle, His —— bell goes tin - kle, tin - kle, Oh his bell goes tin - kle, tin - kle As —— he walks down our street.

110

Un bidon d'eau

French Number Song
Sung to author by Chrissie Paraskevopoulos

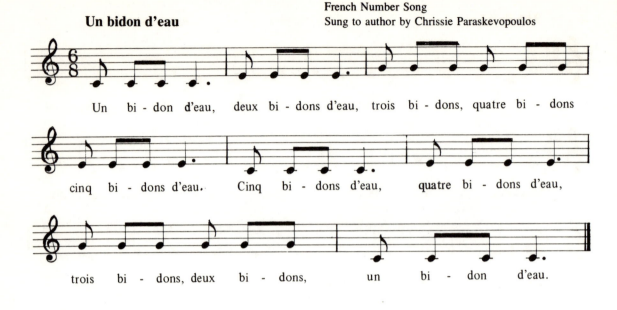

Un bi - don d'eau, deux bi - dons d'eau, trois bi - dons, quatre bi - dons

cinq bi - dons d'eau. Cinq bi - dons d'eau, quatre bi - dons d'eau,

trois bi - dons, deux bi - dons, un bi - don d'eau.

Outdoor Play

The Car

Traditional English Melody
Words and music adapted by Barbara Cass-Beggs

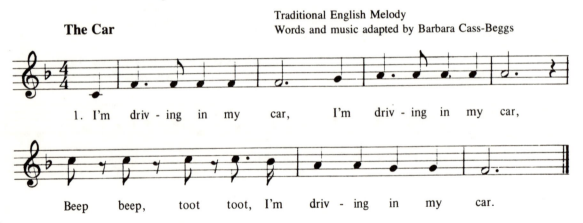

1. I'm driv - ing in my car, I'm driv - ing in my car,

Beep beep, toot toot, I'm driv - ing in my car.

2. I'm driving very fast, etc.
3. I'm driving very slow, etc.
4. The lights are turning red,
   and I must stop my car, etc.,
5. The lights are turning green
   and I can go again, etc.

The Pony

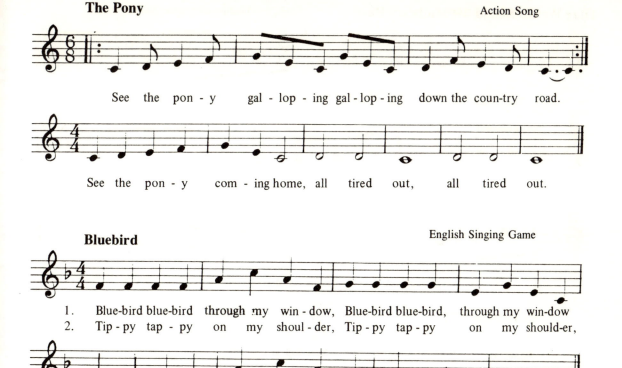

See the pon - y gal - lop - ing gal - lop - ing down the coun-try road.

See the pon - y com - ing home, all tired out, all tired out.

Bluebird

English Singing Game

1. Blue-bird blue-bird through my win - dow, Blue-bird blue-bird, through my win-dow,
2. Tip - py tap - py on my shoul - der, Tip - py tap - py on my should-er,

Blue-bird blue - bird through my win - dow, I love you.
Tip - py tap - py on my shoul - der, I love you.

The children form a circle, raising their arms for windows. A child is chosen to be the bluebird. She flies in and out of the windows and at "tippy tappy" chooses another bluebird, then rejoins the circle. This continues until everyone has had a turn to be a bird.

Here We Go Round the Mulberry Bush

Traditional English Singing Game

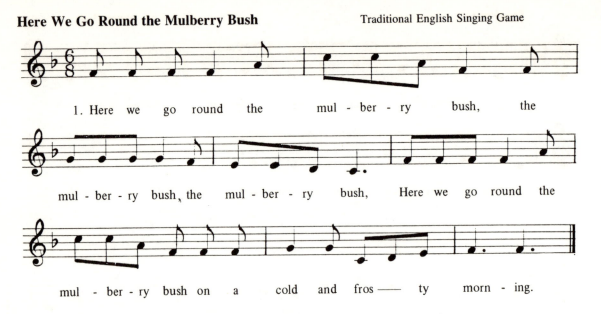

1. Here we go round the mul - ber - ry bush, the mul - ber - ry bush, the mul - ber - ry bush, Here we go round the mul - ber - ry bush on a cold and fros — ty morn - ing.

2. *Dressing.* This is the way we wash our hands, etc.
3. *Gardening.* This is the way we plant our seeds, etc.
4. *Cleaning.* This is the way we brush the floor, etc.

What Shall We Do When We All Go Out

Traditional English Singing Game

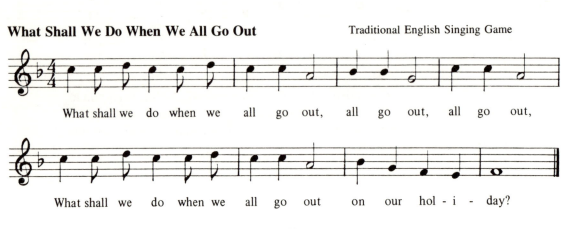

What shall we do when we all go out, all go out, all go out, What shall we do when we all go out on our hol - i - day?

2. We will play with our bouncing ball, etc.
3. We will play with our Teddy bear.

Here We Go Looby Loo

Traditional English Singing Game

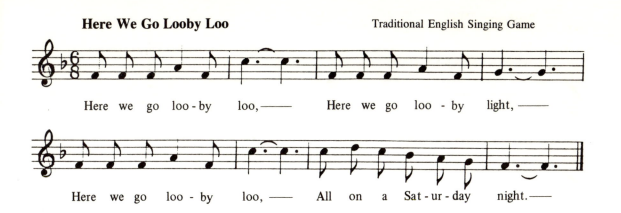

Here we go loo-by loo,——— Here we go loo-by light,———

Here we go loo-by loo, ——— All on a Sat-ur-day night.———

Here We Go Looby Loo
(2nd version)

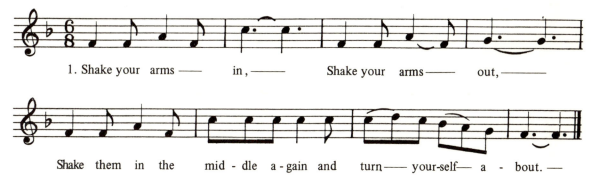

1. Shake your arms ——— in, ——— Shake your arms ——— out,———

Shake them in the mid-dle a-gain and turn——— your-self——— a - bout. ———

2. Shake your foot in,
   Shake your foot out,
   Shake it in the middle again and
   Turn yourself about.

3. Shake your head in, etc.

4. Shake your nose in, etc.

5. Shake your whole self in,
   Shake your whole self out,
   Shake yourself in the middle again and
   Turn yourself about.

Indoor Play

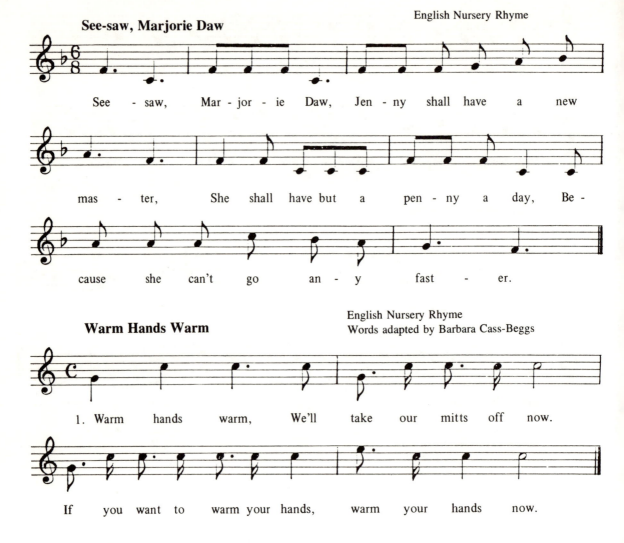

See-saw, Marjorie Daw

English Nursery Rhyme

See - saw, Mar - jor - ie Daw, Jen - ny shall have a new

mas - ter, She shall have but a pen - ny a day, Be -

cause she can't go an - y fast - er.

Warm Hands Warm

English Nursery Rhyme
Words adapted by Barbara Cass-Beggs

1. Warm hands warm, We'll take our mitts off now.

If you want to warm your hands, warm your hands now.

2. Warm feet warm
   We'll take our shoes off now.
3. Clean teeth clean,
   We'll clean our teeth right now.
4. Brush hair brush,
   We'll brush our hair right now.

Hand and Finger Rhymes

Here's a bunny
With ears so funny.
  (raise two bent fingers)
And here's a hole in the ground.
  (make a hole with the fingers of the other hand.)
At the first sound he hears
He pricks up his ears
  (straighten fingers)
And pops right into the ground.
  (pop fingers into the hole)

  (Baby's fingers can be the bunny and mother's the hole, or vice versa.)

~

Put your finger in Foxy's hole,
Foxy's not at home.
Foxy's at the back door
Picking a marrow bone.
  (Form a mound with your hands, making a hole between the
  middle fingers. When the child puts her finger in the hole,
  Foxy gently nips the little finger.)

~

Jack in a box sits so still.
Won't you come out? Yes, I will!
  (Make hands into a fist, thumbs tucked into fingers, then
  pop up the thumbs. Also can be played with a child
  crouching down, then jumping up.)

~

We are little pussy cats
Walking all around.
We have cushions on our feet
And do not make a sound.
  (Make fingers walk around.)

~

Once I saw a little bird
Come hop, hop, hop!
And I cried, "Little bird,
Will you stop, stop, stop!"

I was going to the window
To say "How do you do?"
But he shook his little tail
And away he flew.

Open, shut, and give a little clap.
Open, shut, and put them in your lap.

~

Can you keep a secret?
I don't believe you can.
If you laugh you'll be a gaby,
If you cry you'll be a baby
If you smile you'll be a man.
   (Tickle baby's palm with your finger.)

~

Handy, pandy, sugary candy,
French almond rock.
(Repeat)
   (Put one hand on top of the other, then move the bottom one
   to the top. Baby's and Daddy's hands can join in.
   Gradually bring the bottom hand to the top more quickly.)

~

Bigue bigue beu,
L'est au coin du feu
L'a rien pour son souper
Qu'un p'tit crapaud grillé
Crie saucisse,
Crie saucisson,
Attrap' le!
   (Tickle baby's palm with your index finger. Let baby
   close her hand and catch your finger at ''Attrap' le!'' Then
   let baby tickle your palm, etc.)

~

Le mur se batit,
Le maçon est là,
Une pierre çi,
Une pierre par là.
Ah! Le voilà!
   (Use your hands vertically, placing one above the other with
   each line of the rhyme until baby's eyes are hidden. Take
   them away quickly at ''Ah! Le voilà'')

Creep up to your shoulders high,
Like birds they flutter in the sky,
Like leaves they fall down to the ground,
Pick them up and roll them round.

One is a giant who stamps his feet,
Two is a fairy light and neat,
Three is a mouse who is oh so small,
Four is a great big bouncing ball.
    (Let baby imitate these concepts.)

Two little dickybirds sat on a wall
    (place an index finger on each knee)
One named Peter and one named Paul.
    (raise each finger in turn)
Fly away Peter, fly away Paul.
    (waggle finger as you move arm behind your back)
Come back Peter, come back Paul.
    (return each finger in the same way.)

Pitch Songs

A song to introduce top and bottom doh and soh.

Balloons Up High

Words and music by Barbara Cass-Beggs

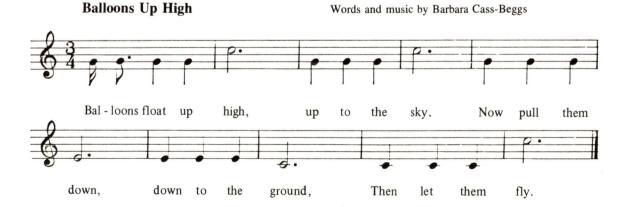

Bal-loons float up high, up to the sky. Now pull them down, down to the ground, Then let them fly.

Throw High, Bounce Low

Words and music by Barbara Cass-Beggs

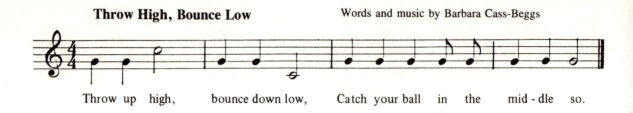

Throw up high, bounce down low, Catch your ball in the mid - dle so.

Rhythm Song

To introduce a slow, moderately slow and quick pulse.

Grandfather's Clock

Words and music by Barbara Cass-Beggs

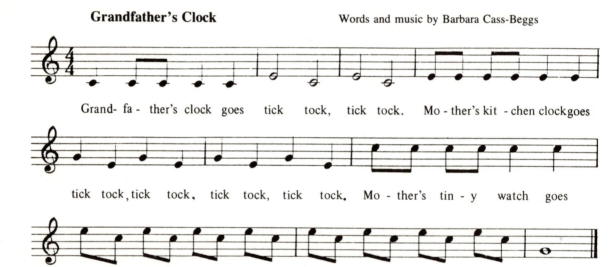

Grand- fa - ther's clock goes tick tock, tick tock. Mo - ther's kit - chen clock goes

tick tock, tick tock, tick tock, tick tock. Mo - ther's tin - y watch goes

tick tock, tick tock, tick tock, tick tock, tick tock, tick tock, tick tock, tick tock, Stop!

Rhymes To Help With Undressing or Dressing

Feetikin, feetikin
When will you gang?
When the night turns short
And the day turns lang,
I'll toddle and gang,
Toddle and gang.

Diddle diddle dumpling
My son John
Went to bed with his trousers on;
One shoe off
And one shoe on,
Diddle diddle dumpling
My son John.

118

9 / Making Your Own Musical Instruments

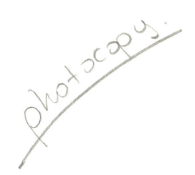

Willie, take your little drum,
With your whistle, Robin, come!
When we hear the fife and drum,
Ture-lure-lu, Pata-pata-pan,
When we hear the fife and drum,
Christmas should be frolicsome.

Burgundian Carol
(English Translation by Percy Dearmer)

Playing musical instruments presents new challenges and helps develop the toddler's dexterity and muscle control. Also, the appearance of the instruments, which you can make quite appealing, increases the child's perceptions of shape and colour. When they are played with other toddlers, they provide an opportunity for co-operative experience.

Different instruments are more suitable at different ages, but all instruments used by the young child *must* be safe to play. They must not have rough or cutting edges, nails, or sharp points. All paint must be non-toxic, and the instrument must be sturdy enough to take rough use without breaking. If you are making a rattle or a maraca, the contents must be securely enclosed or they will surely be put in the child's mouth and swallowed.

Home-made instruments are less expensive than commercial ones and they are fun to make, especially if the whole family gets involved. Making instruments also provides a fine project for a day care centre or a toddler's play group.

With the exception of the largest drum, which appeals instantly to all ages, even to an infant who can only look at it, instruments should be small enough for the baby to hold. Rhythm sticks and claves should be on the small side; variety of tone and attractiveness of shape should be the criteria. Tone blocks are difficult to play unless they have handles; bells, which come in various sizes and shapes, should be easy to hold and not so small that they could be swallowed.

119

Here, then, are a few suggestions for making musical instruments. A book list is included at the end of the section for those who want to make more sophisticated instruments.

Rattles

Rattles or shakers can be made from plastic containers, small tins or plastic egg cups — indeed, any container having a lid which can be securely fastened. The contents can be dried peas, dried beans, rice, tapioca, wheat, maize, small buttons, small pebbles, sand, marbles, beads, washers, or nails; different materials give different sounds, creating variety in pitch and tone quality. Do not use too much filling. Containers may be decorated with paint (non-toxic) or coloured paper securely applied. If you add a handle, make sure that it is firmly attached. For the baby from three months to a year old the containers should be small and brightly coloured.

Bells and Clappers

Small bells need to be firmly attached to some sort of handle; for example, secure four bells with twine to a square of leather which can be screwed on to a brightly enameled dowel rod. A sistrum is simply a stick with bells attached to cross pieces. A large bell can be used on its own; attach a bright cord or strong ribbon to its handle.

Small clappers can be made with cotton thread spools attached to a wood base and enameled with a bright colour. Bells, clappers, and rasps have been used with children as young as three months.

Rhythm Sticks

Lengths of dowelling 6 to 8 inches long and $1/2$ to 1 inch in diameter, enameled in a variety of bright colours, make fine rhythm sticks for the six- to eighteen-month-old child. These can also be used as drum sticks or for hitting tone blocks. By two years the toddler can handle full size rhythm sticks of 12 to 13 inches long and $1/2$ to 3 inches in diameter. Varying lengths and diameters produce different sounds.

120

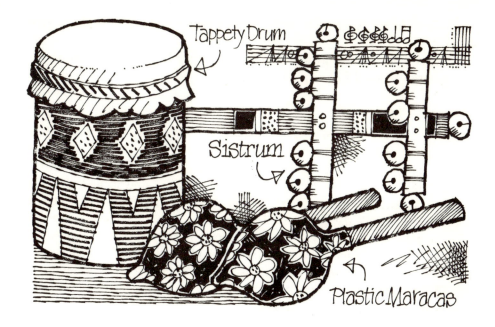

Tappety Drum

Sistrum

Plastic Maracas

Drums

A great variety of drums can be home-made, but perhaps the easiest and sturdiest is made from a round tin box and rubber from a tire's inner tube. The rubber is stretched tightly over the open end of the box, and strong twine threaded through holes punched in the rubber at regular intervals, then secured at the base of the drum to a curtain ring to keep an even tension on the stretched rubber. Paint the drum with gay colours.

Drums can also be made from various sizes of cardboard tubes; the open ends can be covered with parchment, grease-proof paper, or thin rubber sheeting held in place by a strong rubber band secured with glued-on cord, ribbon, or braid. These drums will not last as long as metal ones, but they can be quickly made, and if covered with coloured paper out of which designs have been cut they are very attractive.

Drums can vary in size. A small one will have a soft, high tone; a large drum (which eighteen-month to two-year-old toddlers love) will have a low, louder sound.

A small rubber ball placed on the end of a piece of dowelling makes a good drum stick.

Drums come into their own at the eighteen-month to two-year-old period, but they can be used from six months on.

Maracas

Maracas can be made from plastic lemons or small plastic spice containers covered with papier-mâché, then painted. Any of the ingredients mentioned under rattles may be used to fill them. A handle is a necessity and must be firmly affixed. (Make a hole in the container, insert a small dowel, and glue it in firmly.) Maracas can also be made from electric light bulbs covered with papier-mâché. Once the bulb is completely covered, hit it against a table; this will cause the bulb inside to break and the pieces to rattle whenever it is shaken.

Small gourds which grow in a variety of interesting shapes make lovely maracas or rattles. They can be used as soon as the baby can hold them.

The two-year-old will have fun with a row of variously shaped cooking pans suspended from a clothes line, which she can hit with a rubber hammer. Or you can string a row or two of differently shaped and sized tin cans on twine by making two holes in the tops of each can. These can be hung between chairs or from nails placed across an open cupboard door and two sticks will serve to beat them with. Both these "instruments" can be arranged in a rough scale if graded according to shape and size, and suggest the Javanese or Balinese gamelans.

These and many more elaborate instruments are described in the following books:

Making Musical Apparatus and Instruments for Use in Nursery and Infant Schools by K. Blockside (Nursery School Association of Great Britain and Northern Ireland, 1966)

Making Musical Instruments by Peter Williams (Mills & Boon Ltd., Lively Craft Cards Publication No. 2, distributed by Alfred A. Kalmus, Tonbridge, Kent, England, 1972)

Musical Instruments from Odds and Ends by John Burton (Carousel Books, Transworld Publishers Ltd., London, England, 1976)

Musical Instruments of Africa by B. Warner Dietz and M. Babatunde Olantunji (John Day Co., New York, 1965)

10 / Running a Music Group

Rings on her fingers and bells on her toes,
And she shall have music wherever she goes.

English Nursery Rhyme
("Ride a cock-horse")

If you have enjoyed helping your baby discover music, you may want to take a further step with your two-year-old and organize a small music circle. All you need is a room with space for the young ones to run about in, a record player, and some instruments — as well as a lot of patience and love.

About six or eight toddlers are as many as you will be able to deal with, and even then you will need the help of one or two mothers, including one who has a musical background. It is good to involve some three-year-olds, as they are more accustomed to group activities, and they will enjoy both participating and helping the younger ones.

Because the idea of music groups for babies is a new one, here is an account of one music circle that I enjoyed.

Our music group was kept small so that we could study the individual children. It was made up of a boy of two and five months (Scott), a boy of two (Noah), a girl of twenty-two months (Jill), and three three-year-olds. The group met for one hour a week for twelve weeks. Since it is the children up to two years of age that concern us, I shall not refer to the older ones, who took part in all the activities and did everything slightly better than Noah and Jill but not better than Scott. The three mothers of the younger children participated fully in the first session but did not often attend others, and the children were quite happy on their own.

There were lots of picture books for the children to look at until everyone arrived; then shoes and sometimes socks were taken off and the class was ready to begin.

The first song was one telling them to put the books away in their proper box. Then came an "opening song" during which they all wiggled their toes and fingers, and Scott sang. (After five weeks Noah began singing this song, and by seven weeks Jill joined in with the odd word or two, and obviously enjoyed her participation.) This song was followed by three or four nursery rhymes which were sung and acted out. All three participated in the actions: Scott tried to sing throughout and usually sang part of each song; Noah listened intently and did all the actions; Jill would often get up after one song and run around the room looking at things, but would return to the circle and continue to take part.

After singing, they walked or ran or galloped to the rhythm of a drum. All could walk and run and tiptoe; when we tried a gallop, Scott, who is neat and slight, managed quite a good one; Noah, who is a rather heavy child, walked with a kind of prance; Jill ambled until her attention strayed, then would stop and examine objects in the room. All stopped when the drum said ''stop,'' and they sat down when the drum gave the sit-down signal.

Next came playing the rhythmic patterns of their names on the big drum, which they all loved. Scott and Noah played theirs perfectly, and Jill enjoyed just hitting the drum. Both Jill and Noah were impatient and had to be given several turns.

Since we were all standing up, drum playing was followed by a singing game, ''Ring-Around-A-Rosy.'' This was repeated at least twice, and once the children had reached the ''all fall down'' part, they did not want to get up. Next came a new diversion — rattles, bells, rhythm sticks, or drums (a different instrument each week). Bells or rattles were shaken to music while a song was sung — about rain for the bells and dry leaves for the rattles. As the weeks went by the children were able to shake both bells and rattles more in time with the music. Noah and Jill usually chose their rattles or bells at once, then often wanted to change for a different bell or rattle.

Rhythm sticks were not tried until the sixth week, and to my surprise both Scott and Noah played the three clock sounds exactly (a slow grandfather clock, a faster kitchen clock, and a fast wristwatch). Jill's rhythm was a bit erratic, but she was willing to stop playing when we all stopped. (The first time I suggested that we make the sticks ''run,'' instead of playing a running rhythm on the sticks, she got up and ran around with them.)

At this stage we had a break for juice and cookies, and the children lay on the floor while I sang a lullaby. Noah would usually bury his head in my lap and Jill would cuddle up on my assistant's lap. Scott was quite content to lie down and

124

close his eyes, though if his mother were present (occasionally, we invited the mothers to join us) he would rest on her knee.

The short rest was followed by three more songs and some easy pitch games, using the sol-fa sounds and hand signs. We introduced top and bottom doh and soh and later, me. All children made the correct movements and sang the sounds with us; they loved to sing their names to soh-me. Noah whispered his, but Scott and Jill very quickly sang the correct intervals. In the pitch sounds, Scott and Jill were as good if not better than the three-year-olds.

Pitch games were usually followed by another singing game, "Looby Loo." Apart from the occasional problem of sitting down and holding hands, all went well, with everybody trying to sing. Sometimes instead of singing games we played music which suggested activities the children could take part in at home: gardening, cleaning house, hammering, chopping wood. This provided another outlet for energy and imagination.

They were also introduced to different sounding bells, a variety of drums and, in the eighth week, chime bars. Each child was given a chime bar to be played with a small rubber hammer. I suggested that they hold the chime bar up to their ear after having hit it to find out how long it continued to "sing." They were given only those chime bars which corresponded to the sol-fa sounds they already knew (top and bottom doh, soh and me.) At a later stage, after we had listened to and sung lah and ray, each child was given five chime bars in the pattern of the pentatonic scale and asked to play them very softly, making any patterns they wanted. We also tried giving each child a coloured scarf to wave to the music, but this was not very successful; waving seemed too difficult, and Jill and Noah preferred to drape the scarves over their faces.

From time to time we introduced hand puppets, which came to sing to them, and everyone took turns in holding the puppets, but whereas the "threes" liked to rock the puppets during the lullaby, the "twos" preferred to go to sleep by themselves.

We also provided large-sized scrap books in which we drew balloons and flags related to the pitch songs; rattles and their sound — the sound of pebbles or leaves; bells and their sound — flowers in the wind or falling rain. Scott could draw a circle and straight lines; Jill and Noah made lovely big scribbles and told us what they were drawing (not necessarily what had been suggested). All enjoyed this activity.

125

As the weeks progressed, Jill's attention span increased considerably. She began to sing the songs, and rarely ran around the room on her own. Noah's movements became less awkward; he kept the rhythm better on the rhythm sticks and sang more often. Scott sang all the time on pitch, and unless bored could keep time and play any rhythm.

The three "twos" were more easily distracted than the three "threes" by such things as a ringing phone, a mother's arrival, or a toy that someone had brought from home. The children also needed each activity explained patiently, and yet if the activity did not begin quickly, their attention was lost. For example, Jill could not play the rhythm for the little watch on the sticks until she had told me that "Mummy has a little watch, and where is Mummy?" After her question had been answered satisfactorily, she played the rhythm perfectly.

Moods were very evident: if something had gone wrong before the class began, it took much longer to involve the child completely. Jill, whose mother was expecting another baby, got so excited as the time drew near that it was difficult to hold her attention. Naturally, she wanted all her mother's attention, and we proved very poor substitutes.

We preferred to play or sing all the music, though suitable records could have been used for some of the activities. There was much repetition during the twelve classes, but we varied the subject matter so that things were not repeated in the same way. In rhythm playing we used the drum or rhythm sticks, and the children "played" their names, colours, flowers, animals, what they were wearing, or what they liked to eat. When we played the bells or rattles, we sometimes sang, sometimes played them with accompanying music, and sometimes marched or ran with them. Songs were repeated, but a new one was added every other week, though the opening and closing songs were always the same. The program varied with the mood of the group — an extra lullaby if the children seemed tired, a really energetic exercise if they were particularly lively — but we kept to a pattern, knowing that babies of this age like a sense of order. If we omitted part of the routine, Scott would often notice it — "Why haven't we played the drums?" — and they all asked for "Little Miss Muffett and the spider" every day.

Finding the high, low and middle sounds on the piano was a great favourite; they were ready to listen to each other and say whether Jill was playing the big, low sound of daddy bear's voice or the tiny high voice of baby bear. Loud and soft sounds were the easiest to demonstrate and the easiest for them to distinguish, but they were also able to move and clap quickly and slowly, and towards the close of the classes they could sing with the drum ''stand up'' (soh-doh[1]) and ''books away'' (soh-soh-me). They could also match with their voices the sound of the chime bar that they were playing.

If we consider the variety of imitative musical games that children enjoy, there is no doubt that in the process they are exercising a number of different muscles in a pleasantly relaxed way. To music they can fly like birds or aeroplanes; dance like fairies, ballet dancers or puppets; jump like frogs, rabbits, kangaroos; bounce like big or little balls; rock like a boat, a seesaw, or like a mother rocking her baby; sway like a tree or a flower; creep like a snake or a caterpillar. No toddler will exert herself more than she wants to, and she can always be induced to relax by pretending to be a floppy doll, a balloon with a small hole in it, or a soft, tired kitten. With the ''twos,'' usually a lullaby does the trick.

An hour is a long time to expect two-year-olds to concentrate on one activity, even when the time is broken up with pauses for juice and cookies. The children certainly became tired, both mentally and physically, but they were not bored; there was enough variety of musical activities, and they enjoyed concentrating on each one.

The ideal time to make music with a child is when she desires it and not at a set time, but this is impossible for a class. On the other hand, children enjoy routines for eating, sleeping, and getting dressed, so there is no reason why music should not be part of a routine. Our toddlers knew they were coming to the group to make music and frequently asked their mothers, ''Is it music day today?'' Scott and Jill had older sisters in music classes, and all three mothers were interested in music, though they felt that they did not know much about it.

Such a class unquestionably demonstrates that music can help children with their speech development, muscle co-ordination, sense of pitch, and their ability to co-operate with other children and adults, for example, by taking turns. Most importantly, it helps them to concentrate through listening and to enjoy a happy learning situation in which they can express themselves. It also helps teachers and parents to discover and make the best use of the children's potential.

11 / Suggested Records for Young Children

How many days has my baby to play?
Saturday, Sunday, Monday,
Tuesday, Wednesday, Thursday, Friday,
Saturday, Sunday, Monday.
Hop away, skip away,
My baby wants to play;
My baby wants to play every day.

English Dandling rhyme

Your baby will be more interested in music which involves your participation than in records made for children, and your two-year-old, though she may enjoy the idea of listening to recorded music (particularly if she has her own sturdy player and can put the records on and take them off herself), will not listen for long and still prefers to sing along with you. There are some excellent records made specifically for young children, but they are not always available in the average record shop. If you can interest your local dealer in watching out for new releases for you, it may stimulate him to carry more children's recordings. Here is a short list of useful discs.

BOWMAR RECORDS, 622 Rodier Drive, Glendale, California

Children's Rhythm in Symphony (5.2053)
Rhythm Time (1.023; 2.024)

COLUMBIA RECORDS INC., Educational Division, 799 Seventh Ave., New
    York, N.Y.

A First Record for Children — Dotty Evans, Tom Glazer, Robin Morgan
    (CL 680)
Selections from Tchaikovsky's Nutcracker Suite and The Sleeping Beauty
    (T.W.O. 183)

128

FOLKWAYS RECORDS AND SERVICE CORP., 117 W. 46 St., New York, N.Y.

Adventures in Rhythm — Ella Jenkins (8273)
Animals — Alan Mills (7021)
Birds, Beasts, Bugs and Little Fishes — Pete Seeger (7610)
Call and Response — Ella Jenkins (7308)
Israeli Songs for Children (in Hebrew) — Miriem Ben-Ezra (7226)
More Animals — Alan Mills (7022)
Music Time — Ella Jenkins (3707)
Nursery Days — Woody Guthrie (7208)
Songs to Grow On — Woody Guthrie (7015)

GOLDEN RECORDS: A.A. Records Inc., 250 W. 67 St., New York, N.Y.

Golden Treasury of Music for Children to Dance To (G.L.P. 37)

NONESUCH RECORDS (Explorer Series), WEA Music of Canada Ltd., 1810 Birchmount, Toronto, Ontario.

Flower Dance (Japanese Folk Melodies) (H7.2020S)
The Jasmine Isle (Gamelan Music) (H7.2031)

These two records are suitable for a quiet play period or when the baby is resting.

Voices of Africa (Drums and Voices) (H7.2026)

Parts of this record can be accompanied with percussion instruments or used as a background for vigorous movement.

YOUNG PEOPLE'S RECORDS INC. and THE CHILDREN'S RECORD GUILD, 255 Park Avenue, New York, N.Y.

Let's All Join In (403)
The Neighbor's Band (726)

These records, expecially suitable for the 3-5 age group, can be ordered directly from the company; other titles are also available.

Following is a list of small, inexpensive records which can be ordered directly from the producing companies:

E.M.I. RECORDS. MUSIC FOR PLEASURE LTD., 80 Blyth Road, Hayes, Middlesex, England

Clocks; Church Bells; Farmyard Animals; Domestic Animals; Trains; Aeroplanes and Cars ("sound" records)
My Own Nursery Rhyme Record (MFP 1192) (full size)

PAXTON EDUCATIONAL RECORDINGS, Borough Green, Sevenoaks, Kent, England

Activity Songs (EEP 512)
Finger Play Songs, Set 1 (EEP 507)
Let's Have Fun — Marion Anderson (EEP 545)
Music for Movement, Sets 1-2-4 (E7P 310; E7P313; E7P 319)
Nursery Rhymes and Ring Games (EEP 506; EEP 545)

For mothers who are not familiar with traditional nursery rhymes, these records, with percussion and piano accompaniment, are excellent:

Nursery Rhymes, Sets 1-4 (E7P 301, 302, 303, 308)

ROBIN RECORDS (Educational Rhythms), 86 Newman St., London, W1P.4AR, England

Electronic Music (3 YEG 8762)
La Nursery Ingelbrecht (YEG 8726)
Listen, Move and Dance, arr. Vera Gray (1, YEG 8727; 2, YEG 8728)
Tunes for Children, arr. Roger Fiske and J. P. Dobbs (1, YEG 8575; 2, YEG 8576)

A record meriting special attention is "Lullaby from the Womb" by Dr. Hajime Murookas (Capitol Records) which contains "mother sounds" for the new born baby as well as relaxing music.

12 / Suggested Music for Mothers

Strangely to the brain asleep
Music comes.

John Freeman
(from ''Music Comes'')

I have no uncertainty about the contribution that rhythmical and soothing music make in increasing a baby's sense of security both before and after birth, but when it comes to suggesting specific music for mothers to listen to, I can recommend only certain pieces that have appeal for me, for obviously music selection is a very personal matter.

If you already have strong music preferences and a record library of your own, you will not need my suggestions, but if you rarely listen to music and do not know where to start, my list, which is largely classical, may help you on the way. You may prefer popular music, but do try some of the music listed, if only to add variety, which your baby, too, will appreciate.

When we select a piece of music for listening we are usually influenced by our mood, so I have classified my list by the mood the music suggests to me. I have given the name of the music only and not a specific recording, as you may prefer one artist's recording to another.

Records are expensive, but you do not need a large collection, and by adding a few at a time that you truly enjoy, you will build a record library that will give you pleasure for many years. There are several good record clubs you could join, and many public libraries now have record-lending facilities. Radio programs, too, provide enjoyable music listening, but being able to choose what you want to hear when you want to hear it is important.

We know that music can help subnormal and emotionally disturbed persons. This is because the sounds and vibrations transmitted by the ear to the brain are transformed into emotions and can create favourable attitudes towards the awareness of tension and conflicts, often leading to their resolution.

Thus, music is a more powerful tool than we realize, and because we want our baby to listen along with us it is worth considering the type of music we listen to. Even in its simplest forms music is evocative of sensations, moods and

131

emotions which can affect our sense of security and happiness and either *in*crease or *de*crease our emotional stability. For this reason I have limited my list to "safe" music, music which has form and structure and has stood the test of time.

Besides the pieces listed here there are many other musical areas to be explored: operettas, stage and film musical scores, Gilbert and Sullivan excerpts, choral music, any guitar or lute music, traditional and contemporary folk music, bird songs, even non-music records such as Murray Schafer's "Vancouver Soundscape," which introduces natural sounds of the city and the sea into your living room. The only music I urge you to avoid is that which is noisy and overstimulating, for loudness not only overwhelms content, but when played with the intensity of today's amplification of musical instruments, will in time affect the ability to hear.

So sit down, put up your feet, and listen to music — your choice or mine. Make a note of those titles you particularly enjoy or that you feel have a marked effect on your baby. If you enjoy making your music list half as much as I have enjoyed making mine, you will be in for a happy time.

Restful

Bach — Air on the G String; Prelude No. 1 in C

Beethoven — Piano Sonata, Op. 27, No. 2 ("Moonlight"): first movement; Violin and Piano Sonata No. 5 in F, Op. 24 ("Spring"): first movement

Brahms — Three Intermezzi, Op. 117; Lullaby (song)

Debussy — Suite Bergamasque: Clair de lune

Delius — Fantasy, In a Summer Garden; On Hearing the First Cuckoo in Spring

Grieg — Peer Gynt Suite I: Morning

Humperdinck (arr. Kempe) — Hansel and Gretel Suite

Mendelssohn — A Midsummer Night's Dream: Incidental Music; Violin Concerto in E minor, Op. 64: second movement

Mozart — Quintet in E Flat, K. 452 for Piano and Winds: second movement

Respighi — The Pines of Rome; The Fountains of Rome

Schubert — Piano Trio in B Flat, Op. 99: second movement; Quintet in A for Piano and Strings, Op. 114 ("The Trout"): third and fourth movements

Vaughan Williams — Fantasia on "Greensleeves"

Vivaldi — The Four Seasons: Summer

Thoughtful and Sad

Bach — Harpsichord Concerto No. 5: part two
Chopin — Prelude No. 15 in D Flat ("Raindrop")
Grieg — Peer Gynt Suite I: Asa's Death
Mahler — Symphony No. 2 in C minor: fourth and fifth movements
Rachmaninoff — Piano Concerto No. 2 in C minor: second movement
Saint-Saëns — Carnival of the Animals: The Swan
Schubert — Symphony in B minor ("Unfinished"): second movement

Lively and Happy

Bartók — Concerto for Orchestra: second movement
Beethoven — Violin Concerto in D, Op. 61: third movement; Symphony No. 6
    in F ("Pastoral"): fifth movement
Bizet — L'Arlésienne Suite: March and Theme
Borodin — Prince Igor: Polovtsian Dances
Brahms — Rhapsodies, Op. 79
Britten — Simple Symphony for Strings, Op. 4: first and second movements
Copland — Appalachian Spring (ballet): Rodeo
Schubert — Ecossaise, Op. 189
Schumann — Carnaval, Op. 9

Interesting and Stimulating

Bach — 48 Preludes and Fugues (any); Organ Toccata and Fugue in D minor
Beethoven — Violin Concerto in D, Op. 61: first movement; Symphony No. 3
    in E Flat ("Eroica"): last movement
Debussy — La fille aux cheveux de lin; Prelude à l'apres-midi d'un faune
Elgar — Enigma Variations, Op. 36
Haydn — Symphony No. 101 in D: second movement
Mendelssohn — The Hebrides: Overture
Prokofiev — Romeo and Juliet (ballet): Cushion Dance
Purcell — The Indian Queen: Trumpet Overture
Rimsky-Korsakoff — The Flight of the Bumble Bee
Saint-Saëns — Carnival of the Animals: The Elephant; The Lions
Schumann — Piano Concerto in A minor, Op. 54: first movement

13 / Suggested Reading

In between their outside covers
Books hold all things for their lovers.

Eleanor Farjeon
(from ''The Children's Bells'')

Any list of books related to parent, baby, and music will be endless, for new and useful books are constantly being published, so this list is limited to those that I consider the most important.

Learning About Baby

Birkbeck, A. and M. Moore. *Controlled Childbirth*. Vancouver, B.C.: J. J. Douglas, 1975.

Bowlby, J. *Child Care and the Growth of Love*. Middlesex, Eng.: Penguin Books (Pelican), 1965.

Day B. and M. Liley *The Secret World of the Baby*. New York: Random House, 1968.

Frailberg, S. H. *The Magic Years*. New York: Scribner and Sons, 1959.

Gesell A. and F. Ilg, *The First Five Years of Life*. New York: Methuen, 1950.
_____ and others. *Infant and Child in the Culture of Today*. New York: Harper, & Row, 1974.

Griffiths, R. *The Abilities of Babies*. London, Eng.: University of London Press, 1954.

Isaacs, S. *Intellectual Growth in Young Children*. New York: Schocken, 1966.
_____. *Social Development of Young Children*. London, Eng.: Routledge, 1935.

Leach, P. *Babyhood*. Middlesex, Eng.: Penguin Books, 1964.

Le Boyer, F. *Birth Without Violence*. New York: Alfred Knopf, Inc., 1975.

McDiarmid, N., M. Peterson and J. Sutherland. *Loving and Learning*. Don Mills, Ont.: Longmans Canada Ltd., 1975.

Piaget, J. *The Child and Reality*. London, Eng.: Frederick Muller Ltd., 1974.

Spock, B. *Baby and Child Care*. New York: Hawthorn, 1976.

Understanding and Nurturing Infant Development. Washington, D.C.: Assoc. for Childhood Education, 1976.

Note: Some interesting research projects have demonstrated that an infant as young as a day and a half is conscious of and affected by sound, and although the actual research methods may not concern us, from a musical point of view the projects reveal that infants at this age have a greater sensitivity to sound than has hitherto been recognized.

Valuable information from the medical point of view has also been provided by this type of research, for through sound and the infant's reaction to sound it is possible to distinguish between the healthy infant and the infant with some kind of disorder. (See Author's References, Ch. 2, p. 140, R. Eisenberg: "Auditory behavior in the human neonate" and "Critical age periods and their relation to development disorders of communication.")

Another research finding that can help us discover when the baby is happy and relaxed and perhaps enjoying the music we are playing to her is concerned with the age at which baby can smile. Early smiling used to be attributed to "gas," but this more recent research demonstrates that a baby can smile at birth, and certainly as young as five days old. (See Author's References, Ch. 2, p. 140, M. Tautermannova, "Smiling Infants.")

Introducing and Teaching Music to the Young Child

Aronoff, F. W. *Music in Young Children*. New York: Holt, Rinehart & Winston, 1969.

Birkenshaw, L. *Music for Fun, Music for Learning*. Toronto: Holt, Rinehart & Winston, 1974.

Cass-Beggs, B. *To Listen, To Like, To Learn*. Toronto: Peter Martin Assoc., 1974.

Dalcroze-Jacques, E. *Rhythm, Music and Education*. New York: Putnam, 1921.

Diller, A. and K. Stearns Page. *A Pre-School Music Book*. New York: G. Schirmer, Inc., 1936.

Orff, C. *Orff-Schulwerk Music for Children*. Doreen Hall, trans. London, Eng.: Schott Co. Ltd., 1960.

Richards, M. H. *The Child in Depth*. Portola Valley, Ca.: Mary Helen Richards Institute of Music Education and Research, n.d.

Szonyi, E. *Kodály's Principles in Practice*. London, Eng.: Boosey and Hawkes, 1973.

Suzuki, S. *Nurtured By Love*. New York: Exposition Press, 1969.

Song Books for Children

Buck, Percy, comp. *The Oxford Nursery Song Book*. London, Eng.: Oxford University Press, 1933.

Cass-Beggs, B. *Canadian Folk Songs for the Young*. Vancouver, B.C.: J. J. Douglas Ltd., 1975.

_____, and M. Cass-Beggs. *Folk Lullabies*. New York: Embassy Music Corp., 1969.

Crane, W. *The Baby's Bouquet*. London, Eng.: Pan Books, Piccolo edition, 1974.

_____. *The Baby's Opera*. London, Eng.: Pan Books, Piccolo edition, 1974.

Fletcher, M. I. and M. C. Denison. *The New High Road of Song*. New York: W. J. Gage Ltd., 1950.

Gudin, J., M. C. Maine and J. Brun. *Formulettes pour jouer et chanter*. Paris: Editions Fleurus, 1973.

Landeck, B. *Songs to Grow On*. New York: Edward B. Marks Music Corp., 1950.

Matterson, E. *This Little Puffin*. London, Eng.: Penguin Books (Puffin), 1972.

Panabaker, Lucile. *Lucile Panabaker Song Book*. Toronto: Peter Martin Assoc., 1968.

Simon, Henry W. *A Treasury of Christmas Songs and Carols*. Boston: Houghton Mifflin Co., 1955.

Acknowledgements

I would like to thank the following:

The three mothers whose children attended the music classes for two-year-olds in Vancouver: Gail Owen, Joan Russell, and Penny Geer;

Betty Hyde, Director of Early Childhood Education, Algonquin Community College, Ottawa, and Dr. William Fowler, Ontario Institute of Education, Toronto, for reading the manuscript and providing helpful criticism;

Evy Paraskevopoulos and her daughter Chrissie, for help with the selection of the French songs and rhymes;

Caroline Gibson and her daughter Julia, for additions to the chanting rhymes;

Dr. Desmond Sergeant, Ph.D., G.R.S.M., A.R.C.M., Head of the Music Department, Froebel Institute, London, England, for allowing access to his research library and permitting the use of relevant material;

Dr. R. P. Gannon, M.D., Senior Medical Advisor, Department of Audiology, Workers Compensation Board of B.C., for making time to discuss questions relating to hearing;

Dr. P. Charuhas, M.S.E., Advisor, Department of Audiology, Workers Compensation Board of B.C., for making time to discuss questions on speech;

Michael and Rosemary Cass-Beggs, for reading the manuscript and providing Duncan and Nicholas for observation;

Ruth C-B. Smith for reading the manuscript and providing David Romney for observation;

Mary Termuinde of Vancouver, for photographs of her granddaughter;

Beverly Olandt of Vancouver, for photographs of the class of two-year-olds.

Music Credits

The New Born Baby

"Arroro mi niño" was collected by Lillian Mendelssohn (*Lullabies of the World*, Folkways Ethnic Library, F.E. 4511, New York.)

"Ba Ba Baby" is used by permission of Helen Creighton who collected it from Miss Denny of Eels Ground, N.B.

"Babushka Baio" is a Russian folk lullaby, one version of which can be found in *Songs of the Russian People*, Shreddoll and Smirnova (New York, 1939).

"Bishyby," a Scottish croon, was collected by A. Gilchrist from his grandfather, *Journal of the Folk Song Society* (London), vol. 5, p. 121.

"A Blessing," English folk song, was collected by Cecil Sharp, 1906.

"Bye Baby Bunting," one of many versions of a traditional lullaby, probably came originally from *Tommy Thumb's Song Book*, 1788.

"Do Do" was sung to the author in French by Chrissie Paraskevopoulos.

"Go to Sleep" is a plantation song from Alabama, U.S.A. It was popular in England around 1900 and was sung to the author by her mother.

"Hoe Laat Is't" was collected by Jaap Kunst (*Living Folksongs and Dance Tunes* from the Netherlands, Folkways 3576, New York, 1956).

"Ho Ho Watanay" is used with permission of Alan Mills, who collected it from the Caughnawaga Indian Reservation near Montreal in 1955. The French words printed here are by Evy Paraskevopoulos.

"Hushabye Baby" is set to a musical variation of "Lillibulero," attributed to Henry Purcell. The words are from *Mother Goose's Melodies*, 1765.

"Hush-a-bye birdie" from The Oxford Nursery Rhyme Book, assembled by Iona and Peter Opie

(Oxford University Press, 1955), p. 19, is printed with the publisher's kind permission.

"Hushaby, Don't You Cry" is a traditional American lullaby.

"Rosiçka," a traditional Slovakian melody, was sung to the author by Anne Hruchair of Ottawa.

From Three To Six Months

Unless otherwise noted on the music, all the songs and rhymes in this section are traditional folk songs or nursery rhymes and have been known to the author since childhood. Almost all the English nursery rhymes and finger and toe rhymes in this book can be found in the *The Oxford Nursery Rhyme Book*, assembled by Iona and Peter Opie, and published by Oxford University Press. "Dance to Your Daddy" appears in a collection of Cecil Sharp. Many of the French rhymes in this book are in *Favourite French Folk Songs*, compiled and arranged by Alan Mills (Oak Publications, 1963) or in *Chantons un peu*, selected and arranged by Alan Mills (Toronto: B.M.I., 1961).

From Six to Eighteen Months

The English nursery rhymes and songs in this section were all sung to the author as a child by various members of her family. The French nursery songs are also traditional, as are the finger and body rhymes and chants.

"Sur le dos d'une petite souris" by Adelard Lambert was collected by Marius Barbeau in *Les enfants disent* (Montreal, 1943).

"Toi, toi, toi" has words by Evy Paraskevopoulos set to a traditional French nursery rhyme.

Eighteen Months to Two Years

Almost all of the songs and rhymes in this section are traditional, as are the chants.

"Getting Up Stairs," is from *Leah Jackson Wolford's The Play-Party in Indiana*, edited and revised by W. Edson Richmond and William

Tillson (Indianapolis: Indiana Historical Society, 1959), pp. 153, 54; the words were adapted by Caroline Gibson.

Ruth Crawford Seeger suggested the words for "Mary Wears a Red Dress," "This Is the Way We Put On Our Pants," and "Where Oh Where."

"Tout la haut" was sung to the author by Evy Paraskevopoulos.

The Two-Year-Old

Chrissie Paraskevopoulos sang the words to the French number song "Un bidon d'eau" for Mrs. Cass-Beggs, and Evy Paraskevopoulos suggested the words for "Papillons volez" and "Un deux trois," as well as for the rhymes "Bigue bigue beu" and "Le mur se bâtit."

A slightly different version of "I Went to Visit a Farm One Day" is published in *This Little Puffin* by Elizabeth Matterson (Harmondsworth, England: Penguin, 1969).

"See the Pony" is from *Singing Time* by Satis N. Coleman and Alice G. Thorn, originally published by John Day. Coleman and Thorn suggested words for "Down by the Station," and Marion Anderson provided an idea for the words to "Watch my Dogs."

"The Wheels of the Bus" was originally published by Ginn & Co., Boston, Mass.

The rhymes "Can You Keep a Secret" and "Handy Pandy" were provided by members of the author's family. The rhymes on pages 115 & 117 are courtesy of the Day Nurseries Branch, Dept. of Social and Family Services, Parliament Bldgs., Toronto, Ont.

Author's References

Introduction

Birkbeck, A. and M. Moore, *Controlled Childbirth*. Vancouver, B.C.: J. J. Douglas Ltd., 1974.

Fowler, Dr. W. *Development Methods for Physical Care Routines with Infants*. Toronto: Dept. of Applied Psychology, Ontario Institute for Studies in Education, 1972.

_____ . *Guide for Organization and Supervision of Infants and Pre-School Children*. Toronto: Dept. of Applied Psychology, Ontario Institute for Studies in Education, 1973.

Freud, A. in collaboration with D. Burlingham. *Young Children in Wartime; Infants Without Families*. New York: International Universities Press, 1973.

Harlow, H. F. and M. K. "The effect of rearing conditions on behaviour." *Bulletin of the Menninger Clinic*, no. 26, 1962, pp. 213-224.

Hunt, M. *Intelligence and Experience*. New York: The Ronald Press, 1961.

McQueen, C. M., ed. "Two controlled experiments in music therapy." *British Journal of Music Therapy*, vol. 6, no. 3, 1974.

Michel, P. "The optimum development of musical abilities in the first years of life." *Psychology of Music*, vol. 1, 1973, pp. 14-20.

Pederson, D. R. "The soothing effects of vestibular stimulation as determined by frequency and direction of rocking." ERIC Document Reproduction Service, no. ED 084017.

Piaget, J. *The Child and Reality*. London: Frederick Muller Ltd., 1974.

Pickard, P. M. *The Activity of Children*. New York: Humanities, 1967.

Proielo, D. "Music in Rehabilitation." *British Journal of Music Therapy*, Summer, 1977.

Rheingold, H., J. Gewitz and H. Ross. "Social conditioning of vocalization in the infant." *Journal of Comparative Physiological Psychology* 52, 1959, pp. 68-73.

Sandor, F. *Musical Education in Hungary*. Intro. by Z. Kodály. London, Eng.: Barrie and Rockliff, 1966.

Speigler, D. "Factors involved in the development of pre-natal rhythmic sensitivity." Unpublished Ph.D. Dissertation. Morgantown, West Va.: West Virginia University, 1967.

Stone, L. J., comp. *The Competent Infant*. London, Eng. Tavistock Publishers Ltd., 1974.

Suzuki, S. *Nurtured by Love*. New York: Exposition Press, 1969.

Thompson, J. *Educating Your Baby*. London, Eng.: Oldbourne Book Co. Ltd., 1967.

Tomat, J. H. and C. D. Krutzky. *Learning Through Music for Special Children and Their Teachers*. Merlam-Eddy Co., n.d.

Varo, M. "The musical receptivity of the child and the adolescent." Vol. 1 of the proceedings of the Music Teachers National Assoc., Chicago, 1942.

Young, W. T. "Efficacy of self help program in music for disadvantaged pre-schools." *Journal of Research in Music Education*, vol. 23, no. 2, 1975, p. 99.

Chapter 1: Before Birth

Bench, R. J. "Sound transmission to the human foetus through the maternal abdominal wall." *Journal of Genetic Psychology* 113-114, 1968-69, pp. 85-87.

_____ and P. J. Mittler. "Changes of heart rate in response to auditory stimulation in the human foetus." Abstract, *Bulletin of The British Psychological Society* 20.14.A, 1976.

Cass-Beggs, B. and M. *Folk Lullabies*. New York: Oak Publications, 1969.

Day, B. and M. Liley. *The Secret World of Baby*. New York: Random House, 1968.

Dwornicka, B. and others. "Attempt of determin-

ing the foetal reaction to acoustic stimulation.''
Acta Oto-Laryngologica 47, 1964, pp. 571-74.

Jensen, A. R. ''Pre-natal influence probably the major environmental factor in measuring intelligence.'' *Harvard Educational Review,* June, 1969.

Johansson, B., E. Wedenbergand and B. Westin. ''Measurement of the tone response by the human foetus.'' *Acta Oto-Laryngologica* 57, 1964, pp. 188-192.

Jones, E. G. and E. Ross, *The First Five Years.* London, Eng.: B.B.C., 1976.

''Mother's heart beat as an imprinting stimulus.'' Transcription of the New York Academy of Science, 1124, no. 7, May 1962.

Murphy, K. P. and C. N. Smyth. ''Response of foetus to auditory stimulation.''*Lancet* 1, 1962, pp. 972-73.

Short, E. *Birth to Five.* London, Eng.: Pitman, 1974.

Chapter 2: The New Born Baby

Bower, T. G. R. ''The object in the world of the infant.'' *Scientific American,* Oct. 1971.

Eisenberg, R. and others. ''Auditory behaviour in the human neonate.'' *Journal of Speech and Hearing Research* 7, 1964, pp. 245-69.

_____ and B. J. Penna. ''Critical age periods and their relation to developmental disorders of communication.'' *Journal of Speech and Hearing Research* 5, 1964, pp. 7-11.

Franz, R. L. ''Pattern vision in new born infants.'' *Science Annals* 140, 1963, pp. 296-7.

_____. ''Visual perception from birth, as shown by pattern selectivity.'' *Annals of New York Academy of Science* 118, 1965, pp. 793-814.

Piaget, J. *The Child and Reality.* London, Eng.: Frederick Muller, 1974.

Tautermannova, M. ''Smiling Infants.'' *Child Development* 44, 1973, pp. 701-70.

Chapter 3: The Baby at Three Months

Eisenberg, R. ''The organization of auditory behavior.'' *Journal of Speech and Hearing Research* 13, 1979, pp. 461-64.

Yarrow, L. J. and others. ''Dimensions of early stimulation and their differential effects on infant development.'' *Merrill-Palmer Quarterly* 19, 1972, pp. 205-18.

Chapter 5: From Six Months to a Year

Penfield, W. ''The uncommitted cortex: the child's changing brain.'' *The Atlantic Monthly,* 1964.

Piaget, J. *The Child and Reality.* London, Eng.: Frederick Muller, 1974.

Chapter 6: From Twelve to Eighteen Months

Juliette, A. *Music and the Handicapped Child.* London, Eng.: Oxford University Press, 1965.

_____. *Music Therapy.* London, Eng.: John Baker, 1966.

Chapter 8: The Two-Year-Old

Bachem, A. *Absolute Pitch.* Urbana, Ill.: University of Illinois Dept. of Psychology, 1955.

Beckett, P. and M. P. Haggard. ''The psychoacoustical specification of tone deafness.'' *Speech Perception,* Series no. 2, 1973, pp. 17-21.

Bentley, A. ''Monotones, a comparison with 'normal' singers, in terms of incidence and musical abilities.'' Music Ed. Research Papers, no. 1. London, Eng.: Novello, 1966.

Deutsch, C. P. *Auditory Discrimination and Learning: Social Factors.* New York: New York Medical School, Institute for Developmental Studies, Dept. of Psychology, 1964.

Kirkpatrick, W. C., Jr. ''Relationships between the singing ability of pre-kindergarten children and their home musical environment.'' Unpublished Ph.D. Dissertation, Dept. of Education.

Los Angeles, Ca.: University of Southern California, 1962.

McGinnis, E. "The psychology of musical talent; Seashore's measurements of musical ability, applied to children of pre-school age." *American Journal of Psychology,* vol. 40, no. 3, 1928.

Seashore, C. E. "The measurement of pitch discrimination." Psychological Monograph 53, 1910, pp. 21-60.

Sergeant, Desmond. "The formation of musical concepts." *The Link* (Froebel Institute, London), 1970.

_____. "The measurement of discrimination of pitch." Paper given at 10th Conference on Research in Music Education, University of Reading, Berkshire, Eng., 1969.

_____ and S. Roche. "Perceptual shifts in the auditory information processing of young children." *Psychology of Music,* vol. 1, no. 2, 1974.

_____ and G. Thatcher. "Intelligence, social status and musical abilities." *Psychology of Music,* vol. 2, no. 2, 1974.

Stanton, H. M. "The inheritance of specific musical capacities." *Psychological Journal* 51, 1922, pp. 157-204.

White, B. and J. C. Watts. *Experience and Environment.* Englewood Cliffs, N.J.: Prentice Hall, 1973.

Wynne, V. T. "Absolute pitch in humans; its variations and possible connections with other known rhythmic phenomena." Devonshire, Eng.: Exeter University, 1973.

Index of Music
(First Lines)

Adam and Eve gaed up my sleeve/36
Ainsi font font font/63
A little ball/88
Allons nous promener/83
A Paris, à Paris/41
Arroro mi niño/23
Baa baa black sheep/60
Ba ba bidju bidju ba/18
Baby jump up/108
Balloons float up high/117
Big jet planes are standing in the airport/103
Bigue, bigue, beu/116
Bishyby, bishyby/17
Bluebird, bluebird, through my window/111
Bonjour, bonjour, bonjour à vous/81
Bye baby Bunting/21
Can you keep a secret?/116
Can you kick with two feet?/65
C'est lui qui est allé à la chasse/68
Choo, choo, choo, choo/88
Clap your hands/108
Creep up to your shoulders high/117
Dance-a-baby diddy/47
Dance thumbkin dance/67
Dance to your daddy/46
Diddle diddle dumpling/118
Do do l'enfant do/19
Dormy dormy dormouse/47
Down by the station early in the morning/102
Eeensy weensy spider went up the water spout/106
En bâteau ma mie, ma mie/40
Eye winker, Tom tinker/45
Father, Mother and Uncle John/44
Feetikin, feetikin, when will you gang?/118
Five little kittens all black and white/88
Five little birds without any home/88
Four and twenty white kye/37
Gai, gai, voi le papa/39

Go to sleep, mammy's little baby/24
Go to sleep my darling baby/20
Grandfather's clock goes tick-tock, tick-tock/118
Handy pandy sugary candy/116
Have you seen our pussy cat/108
Hej pade pade Rosiçka/22
Here is baby's tousled head/69
Here is my book, I can open it wide/70
Here's a ball for baby/104
Here's a bunny/115
Here we go looby loo/113
Here we go round the mulberry bush/112
Hickory dickory dock/58
Ho ho watanay/19
Hoe laat is't?/23
Hop, hop, hop, hop my bunny hop/99
Hot cross buns/85
How do you like to go up in a swing?/100
Hush-a-ba birdie, croon croon/27
Hush-a-bye baby on the tree top/18
Hush-a-bye, don't you cry/20
I have a little pony, his name is Dapple Grey/43
I hear thunder, I hear thunder/97
I hold my fingers like a fish/70
I love little pussy/105
I'll touch my chin/69
I'm driving in my car/110
It's blowing, it's blowing, it's blowing all
    around/97
I went to visit a farm one day/104
Jack and Jill went up the hill/61
Jack-in-a-box sits so still/115
J'aime papa/61
Je partis de Levis/71
Knock at the door, peep in/45
Knock at the door, pull the bell/45
L'araignée tickié monte à la gouttière/106
Leg over leg as the dog went to Dover/71
Le mur se bâtit/116
Les menottes sautent, sautent, sautent/82
Let's go to the wood, says this pig/35